Clinical Electrophysiology
A Handbook for Neurologists

Clinical Electrophysiology

A Handbook for Neurologists

Peter W. Kaplan, MB, FRCP

Department of Neurology
The Johns Hopkins University School of Medicine &
Johns Hopkins Bayview Medical Center
Baltimore, MA, USA

Thien Nguyen, MD, PhD

Department of Neurology
The Johns Hopkins University School of Medicine &
The Johns Hopkins Hospital
Baltimore, MA, USA

WILEY-BLACKWELL

A John Wiley & Sons, Ltd., Publication

Blackwell Publishing was acquired by John Wiley & Sons in February 2007. Blackwell's publishing program has been merged with Wiley's global Scientific, Technical and Medical business to form Wiley-Blackwell.

Registered office: John Wiley & Sons Ltd, The Atrium, Southern Gate, Chichester, West Sussex, PO19 8SQ, UK

Editorial offices: 9600 Garsington Road, Oxford, OX4 2DQ, UK
The Atrium, Southern Gate, Chichester, West Sussex, PO19 8SQ, UK
111 River Street, Hoboken, NJ 07030-5774, USA

For details of our global editorial offices, for customer services and for information about how to apply for permission to reuse the copyright material in this book please see our website at www.wiley.com/wiley-blackwell

ISBN: 978-1-4051-85295

A catalogue record for this book is available from the British Library.

Set in 8.5/11 pt Frutiger Light by Aptara® Inc., New Delhi, India
Printed and bound in Singapore by Fabulous Printers Pte Ltd

1 2011

Contents

Preface, viii
Introduction, ix

Part 1: Central Nervous System Disorders

Section A: Altered consciousness: confusion, delirium and unresponsiveness; agitation hallucination and abnormal behavior

1. Diffuse and frontal fast activity—beta, 4
2. Diffuse slow activity—theta, 6
3. Diffuse slow activity—delta, 8
4. Frontal intermittent rhythmic delta activity, 12
5. Occipital intermittent rhythmic delta activity, 14
6. Triphasic waves, 16
7. Low-voltage fast record without dominant alpha frequencies, 18
8. Alpha coma, 20
9. Spindle coma, 22
10. Low-voltage suppressed pattern, 24
11. Burst/suppression, 26
12. Diffuse slowing—toxic encephalopathy—baclofen, 28
13. Diffuse slowing—metabolic encephalopathy—lithium, 30
14. Diffuse slowing—metabolic encephalopathy—hypoglycemia, 32
15. Diffuse slowing—limbic encephalopathy, 34
16. Focal arrhythmic (polymorphic) delta activity, 36

Section B: Periodic patterns of epileptiform discharges, or seizures

17. Pseudoperiodic lateralized epileptiform discharges, 40
18. Bilateral independent pseudoperiodic epileptiform discharges, 44
19. Generalized periodic epileptiform discharges, 46

Part 2: Seizures

Section A: The Diagnosis of confusional events due to seizures

20. Frontal lobe simple and complex partial seizures, 52
21. Temporal lobe simple and complex partial seizures, 54
22. Parietal lobe simple partial seizures, 56
23. Occipital lobe simple partial seizures, 58

Section B: Status epilepticus
24. Complex partial status epilepticus—frontal , 62
25. Complex partial status epilepticus—temporal, 64
26. Simple partial status epilepticus—parietal, 66
27. Simple partial status epilepticu—occipital, 68
28. Generalized nonconvulsive status epilepticus, 70

Part 3: Conditions of Prolonged Unresponsiveness

Section A: Locked-in syndrome, minimally conscious state, vegetative state, and coma: disorders of consciousness and responsiveness
29. Clinical definitions of impaired responsiveness, 76

Section B: Prolonged unresponsive states
30. Locked-in syndrome—brainstem hemorrhage, 82
31. Vegetative state—postanoxia, 84
32. Minimally conscious state—after large, multifocal strokes, 88
33. Catatonia—psychogenic unresponsiveness/conversion disorder, 90
34. Somatosensory evoked potential Prognosis in anoxic coma, 92
35. Somatosensory evoked potential Prognosis in head trauma, 94

Section C: Evoked Potentials in Consultative Neurology
36. Somatosensory evoked potentials in midbrain lesion—absent cortical responses, 98
37. Somatosensory evoked potentials in diffuse cortical anoxic injury—absent cortical and subcortical responses, 100
38. Somatosensory evoked potentials in prolonged cardiac arrest—absence of all waves above the brachial plexus, 102
39. Somatosensory evoked potentials after prolonged cardiac arrest—absence of all responses except cervical N9, 104
40. Somatosensory evoked potentials—median and tibial after traumatic spinal cord injury, 106
41. Visual evoked potentials in worsening vision, 108
42. Brainstem auditory evoked potentials—in worsening hearing, 110

Part 4: Peripheral Nervous System Disease

Section A: weakness and/or respiratory failure in ICU and on the ward
43. Causes of paralysis and respiratory failure in the ICU, 115
44. The clinical evaluation of neuromuscular disorders, 116
45. Laboratory evaluation of neuromuscular disorders, 117

Section B: Segmental weakness and/or sensory loss
46. Evaluation of segmental peripheral neurological disorders, 120

Section C: Respiratory failure/diffuse weakness
47. Amyotrophic lateral sclerosis/motor neuropathy, 122
48. Critical Illness neuromyopathy, 124
49. Brachial plexopathy, 128
50. Femoral neuropathy, 130
51. Sensory neuropathy/ganglionopathy, 132
52. Lumbar radiculopathy, 134

53. Guillain-Barré Syndrome—demyelinating polyneuropathy, 136
54. Myasthenia gravis—neuromuscular junction, 140
55. Myositis—irritable myopathy, 142
56. Statin-induced myopathy—toxic myopathy/myalgia, 146

Part 5: The Casebook of Clinical/Neurophysiology Consults

57. Occipital blindness and seizures—why?, 150
58. Unresponsiveness—coma, vegetative state, or locked-in state?, 152
59. Unresponsiveness—organic or psychogenic?, 154
60. Patient with a frontal brain tumor—psychiatric depression, paranoia, tumor growth, or status epilepticus?, 156
61. Patient with idiopathic generalized epilepsy on valproate—Metabolic encephalopathy or status epilepticus?, 158
62. Unresponsiveness—psychogenic, encephalopathy, or limbic encephalitis?, 160
63. Respiratory weakness—toxic or metabolic?, 162
64. Failure to wean from a ventilator/internal ophthalmoplegia—bulbar dysfunction, neuromuscular junction problem, or polyneuropathy?, 166
65. Progressive sensory loss and painful gait—radiculopathy, toxic or infectious neuropathy, or myopathy?, 170
66. Slowly progressive leg and arm weakness—radiculopathy, plexopathy, ALS, or CIDP/AMN?, 174
67. Progressive thigh pain and leg weakness—radiculopathy, vasculitis, neuropathy, or amyotrophy?, 178

Index, 181

Preface

Clinical Electrophysiology was designed for residents, neurology attendings, and intensive care specialists. It was conceived as a bridging tool that enables the clinical electrophysiological investigation to be tied in with the neurological consultation. This helps the clinician to order the appropriate electrical test, understand the meaning of the interpretation, and then integrate these findings with the clinical question to arrive at a diagnosis. It may further provide information on the differential diagnosis, the prognosis (where warranted), further relevant investigations, and some brief comments on treatment. A brief clinical reference list is included.

In making this portable aid, we placed emphasis on the inpatient clinical setting, giving the appropriate symptoms and signs, and pertinent electrophysiology results that might be found. The discussion that follows is specific to the figure given. Hence, for example, confused patients may have any of a number of EEG findings, but the discussion and prognosis are directed only to the one pattern under discussion, for example, triphasic waves. Diagnostic questions (particularly on chronic conditions) that would largely be encountered in the outpatient clinic, or investigated after patients' discharge, are not included. Hence, chronic neuropathies, palsies, Parkinson's disease, and most genetic conditions are omitted. Similarly, conditions without electrophysiologic relevancies or those warranting other types of tests (CT, MRI, and ultrasound) are not included. Although a comprehensive tome addressing all neurological testing would clearly be useful, it would not be easily portable.

For immediate relevance to neurology consults, we avoided general discussions of the neurological examination, disease entities and electrophysiology in general, as there are a number of excellent books that address these issues in detail. We recommend, of course, supplemental use of these tomes as they are essential to the understanding of clinical neurology.

The book is organized by the presenting neurological problem, for example, confusion, coma, abnormal movements, or difficulty weaning off a respirator, limb numbness, or weakness. Within these topics, there may be some general diagnostic considerations, definitions of terms, but of principal importance, we provide a test result that may be encountered. For example in a comatose patient, we give an EEG showing an invariant alpha frequency pattern. There follows an interpretation of the illustrated finding, differential diagnosis, prognosis, and references. In this way, the "vignette" starts with a clinical problem and reaches a diagnostic, prognostic, or therapeutic end.

Because the handbook is "problem-oriented," it is not a comprehensive treatment of neurologic problems. It is briefer and covers mostly what a hospital clinician might encounter on neurology consultation rounds in a typical year. The last section, however, is a "casebook," which provides several rarer, but classic, clinico-neurophysiological problems. The casebook format provides more clinical information and leaves the reader to test him or herself as the case unfolds. More information on the electrophysiological findings can be found in the respective section in the handbook.

Please use the book, if helpful, in wording your consults and in providing references. Do give us feedback into any shortcomings and major areas that we failed to include. We hope you find it a useful aide-memoire as you address clinical challenges.

Peter W. Kaplan, MB, FRCP
Thien Nguyen, MD, PhD

Introduction

We have designed this handbook to accompany you on your rounds. We believe that the handbook works best in the "middle step" of the neurology consultation process. In the first step, historical data are collected and an examination is performed to arrive at an opinion, possibly then suggesting complementary tests. If electrophysiological tests are requested, it is at the next step that the handbook is helpful in addressing the significance of the findings, the differential diagnosis, prognosis, and in providing some brief therapeutic directions. In the final step, a concluding opinion can then be formulated. In other cases, the handbook can be used to review the meaning of a particular test result that has already been received, so as to be able to provide further information to the patient's treating physicians.

Too often, the nature and significance of test results can remain uncertain: do they represent a "red herring"? Are they helpful in eliminating or confirming a particular diagnosis among many? What do they tell us about prognosis?

Standard textbooks abound to help with taking the history of a neurological complaint, performing physical examinations, or discussing the many disorders that can be diagnosed. Other texts may discuss in detail the techniques and interpretation of EEG, evoked potentials, NCVs, and electromyography. The handbook bridges the gap between the electrophysiological laboratory and the bedside.

PART 1
Central nervous system disorders

Section A: Altered consciousness: confusion, delirium, and unresponsiveness; agitation, hallucination, and abnormal behavior

These are some of the "altered states" that prompt neurology consults. Patient problems rather than specific, prepackaged "diagnoses" generate consults. Hence, clinical training rather than standard texts is the major source of learning the physician's approach to managing *problem-oriented* questions.

Unfortunately, the causes (or diagnoses) underlying a particular complaint are legion––consider the potential causes of "dizziness," for example, low blood pressure or neurilemmoma, migraine or brainstem stroke, low blood sugar or otolith disease, and multiple sclerosis or Meniere's disease.

Clearly the constellation of symptoms and signs (and those absent) from the patient's description of clinical features (the syndrome) will pare down the possibilities and direct the diagnostic evaluation and investigation. Excellent texts are available that can address "lists" of probable alternatives to particular complaints. Maybe the future will lie in the use of a palm-held computer into which the complaint/symptom will be logged, followed by associated (or not) clinical features, resulting in the generation of a "probability list," which can be used even while one is rounding on patients.

In this section, we address certain states of altered consciousness or behavior that fall short of coma. Locked-in states, minimally conscious states, akinetic mutism, and vegetative states are a different order of "unresponsiveness," and are found in their own section further on. Those examples contained here involve acute or subacute global diminution in the level of consciousness, vigilance, memory, and cognitive processing in keeping with encephalopathies ("altered mental status") or "acute confusional states" due to toxic/metabolic, infectious, or ictal disturbances.

Some definitions in current use are as follows:

Delirium: An acute alteration in cognitive function with impaired short-term memory, sleep cycle inversion, sometimes with increased motor activity in the form of agitation and tremulousness (think withdrawal or delirium tremens), often with amnesia.

Confusion: A general term that usually needs further definition. Often, however, it is used to refer to a state of impaired language output, orientation, the ability to follow commands and to retain information.

Altered mental status: This could subsume the above. Also a non-specific term, which could apply to psychosis, coma, or dementia. It also needs further specification.

Encephalopathy: A Greek-derived term for diffuse brain dysfunction––also non-specific. But then globally confused patients are often perforce "nonspecifically" cognitively impaired (a clue in itself).

Or there may be a clinical question at the outset: Is this nonconvulsive status epilepticus (NCSE)? This is specific and provable one way or the other. One might consider the variety of clinical features seen with NCSE and obtain an EEG.

So where to go? Once the probable type of higher cortical disturbance has been tested, for example, with a mini-mental status examination, more detailed testing of the patient's orientation, language, memory, ability to follow commands, to interpret events (the "cookie thief" picture), and then a probability list of diagnoses can be produced. This might include a consult with the following:

> ***Possible toxic/metabolic encephalopathy. Suggest the exclusion of systemic infection in this patient with chronic diminished tolerance to the many causes of encephalopathy (e.g. cerebral atrophy; dementia). Consider also investigation of ictal/post-ictal possibilities (with an EEG).***

If in the course of investigating altered consciousness or abnormal behavior in a patient, the EEG reveals an epileptiform abnormality, turn then to the section on seizures (Part 2) for further electroclinical correlations and suggestions.

The easier questions to answer are often those centered on a request for *prognosis*. In particular instances such as after anoxia, "ball-park" answers can be provided, or even some highly exact ones. For example, the prognosis in a lethargic patient 3 days after CRA can be given with much support from the literature, and from EEG and SSEPs (somatosensory evoked potentials). For these types of questions and for those patients in coma, locked-in states, and vegetative states, please refer to Part 3 on these disorders. A brief overview on prognosis and evaluation can also be found in the section on Evoked Potentials in Consultative Neurology.

1. Diffuse and frontal fast activity—beta

MICU, CICU, NICU, SICU, WARD, ER

CLINICAL CORRELATES: A patient may have been referred to the electrophysiology laboratory for one of several clinical reasons, and the EEG reveals medium to high-voltage diffuse beta frequencies. In a patient with little history, it would suggest drug intoxication and the need for a toxin screen. The patient may be normal, drowsy, or rarely agitated.

ETIOLOGY: Benzodiazepine, chloral hydrate, or barbiturate treatment or intoxication. Occasionally, sedative withdrawal states. With high medication doses, the patient may be sedated to the point of unarousablility (beta coma, usually >30 μV on EEG). It can occur with brainstem injury [4].

CLINICAL EVALUATION: Record all medications to which the patient has access. Look for medication/sedative effects; alternately, the patient may be agitated rarely with delirium.

ANCILLARY TESTING: Toxin screen for barbiturates or benzodiazepines. MRI of brainstem structures.

DIFFERENTIAL DIAGNOSIS: For the EEG pattern, it may occur with benzodiazepines, barbiturates, sedative withdrawal, childhood mental retardation and cerebral palsy, brainstem injury.

PROGNOSIS: There is little dependable literature on the significance of this finding. The prognosis/reversibility, when this is due to medications, is excellent. In children there is a report of continuous beta spindling in cerebral palsy and mental retardation (extreme spindles). The spindle beta patterns are associated with a good prognosis regardless of etiology, with the exception of children not on barbiturates or benzodiazepines.

Clinical Electrophysiology. By © Peter W. Kaplan and Thien Nguyen.
Published 2011 Blackwell Publishing Ltd.

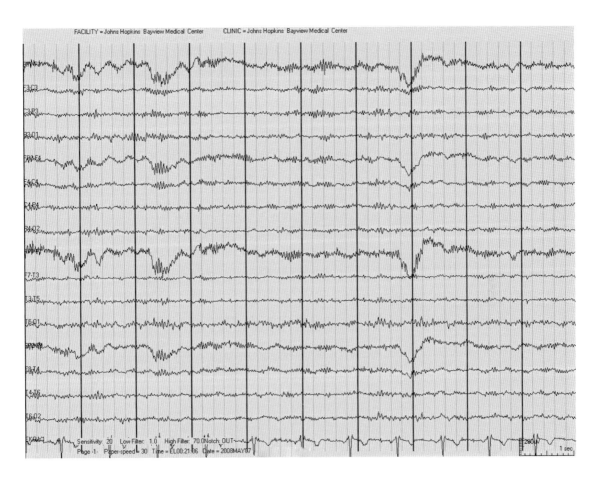

This EEG shows a medium- to high-voltage diffuse fast beta pattern. In this case, it is prominent anteriorly, particularly in light sleep and following arousal. Occasionally, it may show a spindling pattern. On EEG, in general, there are beta frequency bands typically seen at 18–25 Hz, less frequently at 14–16, and in one report at 35–40 Hz. It is considered high voltage when it exceeds 25 µV [1–4]. It was originally, probably incorrectly, believed to be associated with epilepsy, minimal brain dysfunction, dyslexia, hyperactivity, or other behavioral dysfunction. Conversely, this pattern is typical of a medication effect.

REFERENCES:

1. Frost JD, Carrie JRG, Borda RP, Kellaway P. The effects of Dalmane (flurazepam hydrochloride) on human EEG characteristics. *Electroencephalogr Clin Neurophysiol* 1973; 34:171–175.
2. Kellaway P. Orderly approach to visual analysis: Elements of the normal EEG and their characteristics in children in adults. In: Ebersole JS, Pedley TA (eds.), *Current Practice of Clinical Electroencephalography*, 3rd edn. Philadelphia, PA: Lippincott/Williams and Wilkins 2003;100–159.
3. Kellaway P. The development of sleep spindles and of arousal patterns in infants and their characteristics in normal and certain abnormal states. *Electroencephalogr Clinc Neurophysiol* 1952;4:369.
4. Otomo E. Beta activity in the electroencephalogram in cases of coma due to acute brainstem lesion. *J Neurol Neurosurg Psychiatry* 1966;29:383–390.

2. Diffuse slow activity–theta [1–4]

Acute encephalopathies—frequently the elderly, multiorgan failure. Static encephalopathies, mild diffuse cortical dysfunction.

CLINICAL CORRELATES: Psychomotor slowing, confusion, clouding of sensorium. Brainstem function is intact.

ETIOLOGY: In the ICU, causes typically include toxic and metabolic dysfunction, and systemic infection. Often seen in elderly patients with cerebral atrophy with the above causes, as well as in dementias, static encephalopathies, mental retardation, and learning disability.

CLINICAL EVALUATION: Higher cortical function, general neurological examination.

ANCILLARY TESTING: CT or MRI may show subcortical atrophy; evidence of head injury; chronic encephalopathy. Test for organ failure—hepatic, renal, respiratory, or other organ dysfunction.

DIFFERENTIAL DIAGNOSIS: From the EEG perspective, check that the patient is not just drowsy or asleep during this EEG segment (normal drowsy pattern), and ensure that the EEG recording contains adequate noxious stimuli to ensure full arousal during the EEG.

PROGNOSIS: Due to static encephalopathy, it reflects a chronic state of cortical dysfunction and has no particular prognostic import. If seen with organ dysfunction, then the electroclinical picture may be reversible. Even after anoxia, patients with this theta pattern often improve clinically and on EEG [3, 4].

Clinical Electrophysiology. By © Peter W. Kaplan and Thien Nguyen.
Published 2011 Blackwell Publishing Ltd.

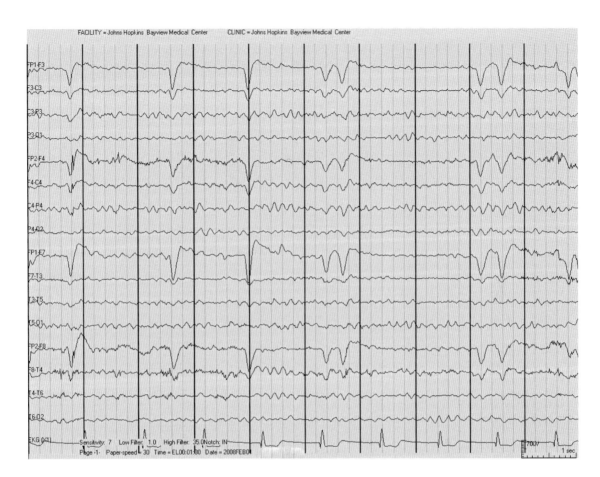

FACILITY = Johns Hopkins Bayview Medical Center   CLINIC = Johns Hopkins Bayview Medical Center

This EEG shows widespread theta activity. There is variable intrusion of alpha and delta frequencies; alpha can be seen with maximal arousal. The eye blink artifact seen every several seconds bifrontally indicates the awake state of the patient. Diffuse theta is onlyless frequent than other EEG patterns seen in confusion/encephalopathic states (possibly due to ascertainment bias).

REFERENCES:

1. Chatrian G-E, Turella GS. Electrophysiological evaluation of coma, other altered states of diminished responsiveness and brain death. In: Ebersole JS, Pedley TA (eds.), *Current Practice of Clinical Electroencephalography*. Philadelphia, PA: Raven Press 2003:405–462.
2. Gloor P, Kalabay O, Giard N. The electroencephalogram in diffuse encephalopathies: EEG correlates of grey and white matter lesions. *Brain* 1968;91:779–802.
3. Silverman D. Retrospective study of the EEG in coma. *Electroencephalogr Clin Neurophysiol* 1963;15:486–503.
4. Yamashita S, Morinaga T, Ohgo S, et al. Prognostic value of EEG in anoxic encephalopathy after CPR. Relationship among anoxic period, EEG grading and outcome. *Intern Med* 1995;34:71–76.

3. Diffuse slow activity—delta [1–3]

MICU, CICU, NICU, SICU, WARD, ER

Seen in elderly patients with multifactorial causes, sub-cortical white matter cerebral atrophy, after closed head trauma. Occasionally occurs with drugs.

CLINICAL CORRELATION: Patients are often deeply ob-tunded. They may have significant brainstem compro-mise, but not invariably.

ETIOLOGY: Young patients with severe metabolic dys-function, deep mid-line lesions, and those of the corpus callosum.

CLINICAL EVALUATION: General neurological examina-tion. Glasgow Coma Scale.

ANCILLARY TESTING: CT or MRI may show subcortical lesions or atrophy; evidence of head injury. Consider SSEPs (somatosensory evoked potentials) for prognosis after trauma. If toxicity is suspected and no other history available, consider drug/toxin screen.

DIFFERENTIAL DIAGNOSIS: From the EEG perspective, only an atypical Stage 4 sleep pattern occasionally resem-bles this pattern. Ensure that the EEG recording contains adequate noxious/arousal stimuli to exclude sleep as an explanation.

PROGNOSIS: There is little dependable literature on out-come, probably because of ascertainment bias. Progno-sis depends on the etiology. Reversible metabolic/organ failure causes have the best prognosis. There is a re-port of complete recovery after drug overdose [4]. With head injury, normal outcomes are less frequent. Se-rial EEGs over time may provide indications of recovery and allow monitoring for subclinical seizures after head trauma.

Clinical Electrophysiology. By © Peter W. Kaplan and Thien Nguyen.
Published 2011 Blackwell Publishing Ltd.

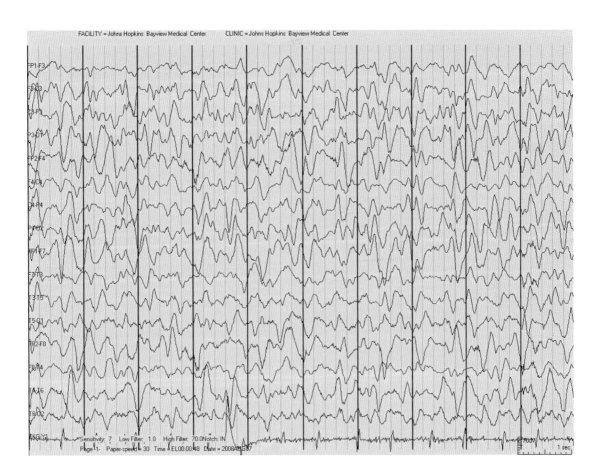

This EEG shows widespread, arrhythmic delta activity at 1–4 Hz (as well as theta and alpha frequencies) over all brain regions. There is relatively little spontaneous variability or reactivity to stimuli. This pattern is surprisingly less common than many other EEG patterns of deep coma.

The second EEG example shows more pervasive slow 0.5- to 4.0-Hz delta activity and lesser amounts of theta activity. The high-frequency filter was set at 15 Hz to minimize muscle artifact in the figure.

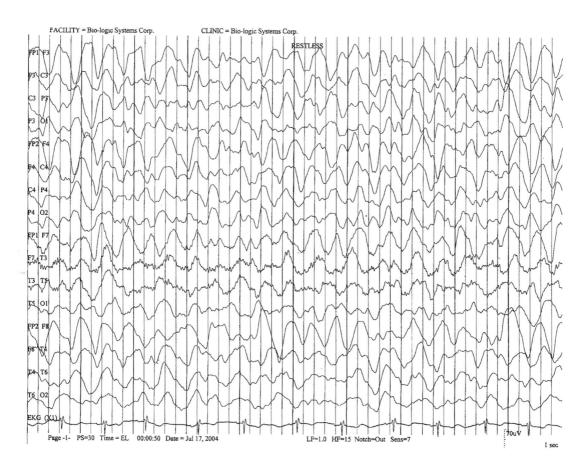

REFERENCES:

1. Chatrian G-E, Turella GS. Electrophysiological evaluation of coma, other altered states of diminished responsiveness and brain death. In: Ebersole JS, Pedley TA (eds.), *Current Practice of Clinical Electroencephalography*. Philadelphia, PA: Raven Press 2003;405–462.

2. Gloor P, Kalabay O, Giard N. The electroencephalogram in diffuse encephalopathies: EEG correlates of grey and white matter lesions. *Brain* 1968;91:779–802.

3. Silverman D. Retrospective study of the EEG in coma. *Electroencephalogr Clin Neurophysiol* 1963;15:486–503.

4. Blume WT. Drug effects on EEG. *J Clin Neurophysiol* 2006;23:306–311.

4. Frontal intermittent rhythmic delta activity [1–5]

Seen in elderly patients with multifactorial causes: cerebral atrophy, dementia, and intercurrent infection.

CLINICAL CORRELATION: Patients are often lethargic or confused, disoriented, but usually conversant and can follow motor commands; myoclonus and seizures are unusual. The patient localizes to pain and brainstem reflexes are usually intact. This EEG pattern is usually seen as alpha activity and wakefulness diminishes.

ETIOLOGY: Concurrent metabolic and infectious problems are frequent [1–5]. Of 68 patients, 78% had hypertension, diabetes, or renal insufficiency [5]. One-third to half of the patients had both renal failure and hyperglycemia with background theta activity; most patients had some cerebrovascular disease and were awake [5]. In children, it was previously thought to indicate increased pressure around the third and fourth ventricles.

CLINICAL EVALUATION: Examine cognitive function, test for neck stiffness, external evidence of trauma, fetor, or dehydration.

ANCILLARY TESTING: Electrolytes and CT/MRI for cerebral atrophy. Consider obtaining a chest x-ray, urine, and blood cultures to look for infection.

DIFFERENTIAL DIAGNOSIS: FIRDA (frontal intermittent rhythmic delta activity) may be mistaken for an eye movement artifact. Gently preventing eye movements during the EEG or use of eye movement EEG montages can differentiate between the two. Use eye leads above and below the eyes.

PROGNOSIS: Largely depends on the underlying cause; may be of value if etiology is known [2–5]. There is a good prognosis with urinary tract infections and reversibly toxic drugs. Prognosis is less favorable with the less reversible organ failures (hepatic) and systemic infections [4]. Given its demographic in aged patients, the overall prognosis is that of underlying conditions.

TREATMENT: The underlying acute and chronic conditions, for example, dementia and intercurrent infection.

Clinical Electrophysiology. By © Peter W. Kaplan and Thien Nguyen.
Published 2011 Blackwell Publishing Ltd.

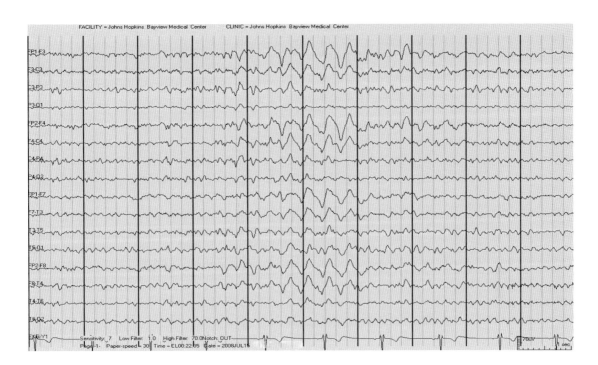

This EEG shows runs of frontal intermittent delta activity with preservation of waking background alpha and theta frequencies. It usually appears at 2–4 Hz and is seen synchronously and symmetrically. Eye leads placed below the eyes can differentiate eye movement artifact from frontal (brain) slowing.

REFERENCES:

1. Chatrian G-E, Turella GS. Electrophysiological evaluation of coma, other altered states of diminished responsiveness and brain death. In: Ebersole JS, Pedley TA (eds.), *Current Practice of Clinical Electroencephalography*. Philadelphia, PA: Raven Press 2003;405–462.

2. Fariello RG, Orrison W, Blanco G, Reyes PF. Neuroradiological correlates of frontally predominant intermittent rhythmic delta activity (FIRDA). *Electroencephalogr Clin Neurophysiol* 1982;54:194–202.

3. Alehan F, Dabby R, Lerman-Sagie T, Pavot P, Towne A. Clinical and radiologic correlates of frontal intermittent rhythmic delta activity. *J Clin Neurophysiol* 2002;19:535–539.

4. Daly D, Whelan JL, Bickford RG, Maccarty CS. The electroencephalogram in cases of tumors of the posterior fossa and third ventricle. *Electroencephalogr Clin Neurophysiol* 1953;5:203–216.

5. Watemberg N, Alehan F, Dabby R, Lerman-Sagie T, Pavot P, Towne A. Clinical and radiologic correlates of frontal intermittent rhythmic delta activity. *J Clin Neurophysiol* 2002;19:535–539.

5. Occipital intermittent rhythmic delta activity [1–5]

WARD, PEDs, OUT Pt

Occasionally seen in pediatric patients with a history of generalized seizures.

CLINICAL CORRELATES: This pattern exists almost exclusively in children. The patient is interactive on arousal.

At the time of EEG, most patients have had a tonic–clonic seizure leading to the referral. During the EEG, patients are usually awake or drowsy, or less frequently asleep [3]. There is often a past history of childhood absences [1,4,5], but recent data indicate an association with localization-related epilepsies [3].

ETIOLOGY: It has been reported with salmonella, Huntington disease, and subacute sclerosing panencephalitis [3], and may occur in Angelman syndrome.

CLINICAL EVALUATION: Take a careful history for seizures. Mean age 8 years (3–16 years).

ANCILLARY TESTING: The brain MRI is normal.

PROGNOSIS: Children whose EEGs contain 3/second spike-and-wave as well as occipital intermittent rhythmic delta activity (OIRDA) may remit within 10 years in more than 50% of cases, and not manifest tonic–clonic seizures; those without OIRDA, but with photoparoxysmal EEG responses, rarely remit spontaneously (6%), and more frequently have convulsions.

TREATMENT: Patients with seizures can benefit from antiepileptic drugs.

Clinical Electrophysiology. By © Peter W. Kaplan and Thien Nguyen.
Published 2011 Blackwell Publishing Ltd.

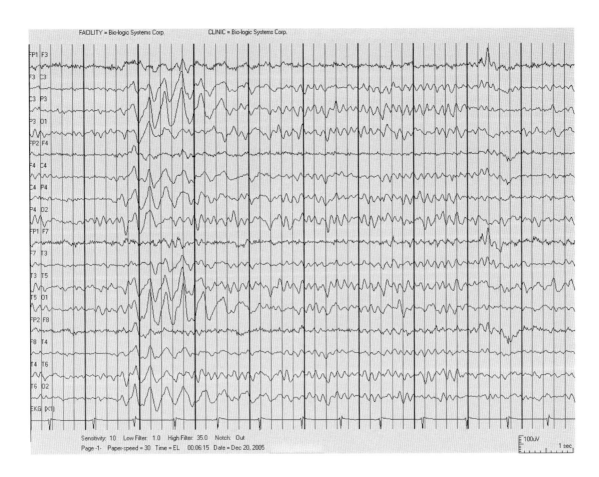

This EEG shows runs of OIRDA with preservation of waking background alpha and theta frequencies. It usually occurs at 2–4 Hz, synchronously and symmetrically with some waxing and waning. It is seen in awake and drowsy recordings of EEG. The background is usually alpha, but may be theta in about a quarter of patients [1]. Half the studies also have focal, concomitant epileptiform discharges. Rarely, OIRDA is brought out by hyperventilation and can co-occur with frontal intermittent rhythmic delta activity (see this rhythm).

REFERENCES:

1. Loiseau P, Pestre M, Dartigues JF, Commenges D, Barberger-Gateau C, Cohadon S. Long-term prognosis in two forms of childhood epilepsy: Typical absence seizures and epilepsy with rolandic (centrotemporal) EEG foci. *Ann Neurol* 1983;13:642–648.
2. Daly DD, Markand ON. In: Daly DD, Pedley TA (eds.), *Current Practice of Clinical Electroencephalography*, 2nd edn. New York: Raven Press 1990;335–370.
3. Watemberg N, Linder H, Dabby R, Blumkin L, Lerman-Sagie T. Clinical correlates of occipital intermittent rhythmic delta activity (OIRDA) in children. *Epilepsia* 2007;48:330–334.
4. Riviello JJ, Foley CM. The epileptiform significance of intermittent rhythmic delta activity in childhood. *J Child Neurol* 1992;7:156–160.
5. Gullapalli D, Fountain NB. Clinical correlation of occipital intermittent rhythmic delta activity. *J Clin Neurophysiol* 2003;20:45–51.

6. Triphasic waves [1–7]

MICU, CICU, NICU, SICU, WARD, ER

Seen with toxic/metabolic illness, often with infection and cerebral/subcortical atrophy.

CLINICAL CORRELATES: Patients are usually lethargic; myoclonus and seizures are unusual. The eyes are open or closed, may open to stimuli. The patient is confused, may be able to speak, but is somnolent. In lighter coma, the patient can follow commands, localize to pain, and have intact brainstem reflexes.

ETIOLOGY: Concurrent metabolic and infectious problems are frequent: hepatic failure, uremia, systemic infection, hyperosmolarity, hypoxia, and hypoglycemia [2–6]. Triphasic waves (TWs) are seen with drug toxicity, for example, lithium, cefepime, baclofen, ifosfamide, levodopa, metrizamide (controversy whether this is NCSE), valproate (with or without raised ammonia), serotonin syndrome, Creutzfeldt-Jakob disease, Alzheimer's disease [2–6].

CLINICAL EVALUATION: In nontraumatic coma, examine cognitive function, test for neck stiffness, look for hepatic fetor, and look for systemic evidence of liver insufficiency (spider naevi, caput medusae, palmar erythema, leukonychia).

ANCILLARY TESTING: Electrolytes, ammonia level, liver profile, toxin screen, and MRI for white matter disease.

DIFFERENTIAL DIAGNOSIS: TWs are blunter and usually of lower frequency than the discharges of nonconvulsive status epilepticus (NCSE). TWs may increase (rarely decrease) with arousal. Background activity can be present with either TWs or NCSE. TWs resolve with benzodiazepines, but the patient fails to improve. Fifty-nine percent of patients with TWs may have nonmetabolic encephalopathies [2].

PROGNOSIS: This largely depends on the underlying cause; the EEG may be of prognostic value if the etiology is known [2–6]. There is a good prognosis with urinary tract infections, reversibly toxic drugs and hyperammonemia in patients on valproate. The prognosis is less favorable with less reversible organ failure (hepatic) and systemic infections [4]. There is a poor prognosis after anoxia [6]. Given its demographic in aged patients, the overall prognosis (from all causes) is poor with a 77% mortality [3]. In 100 patients with severe liver disease, 45 died within 1 week before the advent of liver transplants [7].

TREATMENT: If NCSE is suspected as a differential diagnosis, then a trial of lorazepam 2–4 mg may improve NCSE clinically and either on EEG; benzodiazepines may worsen encephalopathies.

Clinical Electrophysiology. By © Peter W. Kaplan and Thien Nguyen.
Published 2011 Blackwell Publishing Ltd.

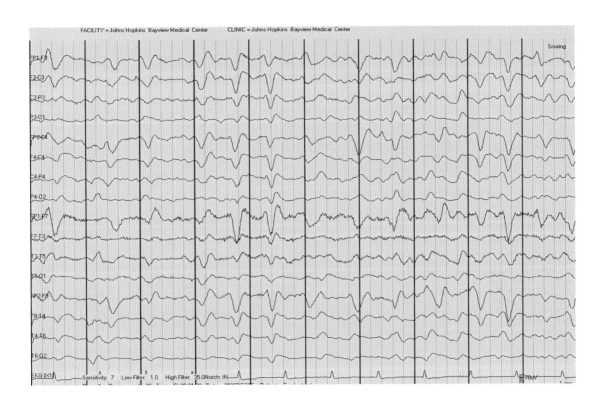

This EEG shows generalized TWs, typified by a blunted or small upgoing (negative) first phase, rapid descending dominant (positive) second phase, less steep, ascending third phase. It is best seen in a referential montage and often brought out by arousal. The frequency of TWs is 1.5–2.5 Hz, of moderate to high amplitude (100–300 µV); the activity is seen in clusters. There is often theta/delta background activity. TWs are often dominant anteriorly, with an anteroposterior lag on a referential montage [2]. The background is slower if seen with hepatic insufficiency. Toxic and metabolic causes cannot be distinguished on EEG [2].

REFERENCES:

1. Bickford RG, Butt HR. Hepatic coma: The EEG pattern. *J Clin Invest* 1955;34:790–799.

2. Sundaram MB, Blume WT. Triphasic waves: Clinical correlates and morphology. *Can J Neurol Sci* 1987;14:136–140.

3. Bahamon-Dussan JE, Celesia GG, Grigg-Damberger MM. Prognostic significance of EEG triphasic waves in patients with altered state of consciousness. *J Clin Neurophysiol* 1989;6:313–319.

4. Young GB, Bolton CF, Archibald YM, Austin TW, Wells GA. The EEG in sepsis-associated encephalography. *J Clin Neurophysiol* 1992;9:145–152.

5. Blume WT. Drug effects on EEG. *J Clin Neurophysiol* 2006;23:306–311.

6. Yamashita S, Morinaga T, Ohgo S. Sakamoto T, Kaku N, Sugimoto, S, Matsukura S. Prognostic value of EEG in anoxic encephalopathy after CPR: Relationship among anoxic period, EEG grading and outcome. *Int Med* 1995;34:71–76.

7. MacGillivray BB. The EEG of liver disease. In: Remond CA (ed.), *Handbook of Electroencephalography and Clinical Neurophysiology*, Vol. 15. Amsterdam: Elsevier 1976;77–87.

7. Low-voltage fast record without dominant alpha frequencies [1]

SICU, MICU, NICU

Seen after head trauma or in alcohol abuse. May be a normal variant.

CLINICAL CORRELATES: The patient may be cognitively normal. Conversely, there may be confusion or lethargy.

ETIOLOGY: Head trauma, normal variant, hydrocephalus, alcoholism.

CLINICAL EVALUATION: General neurological examination. Check for history of closed head trauma, bilateral subdural, epidural, or scalp fluid collections. Ask after a history of alcoholism. Smell for alcohol fetor.

ANCILLARY TESTING: CT or MRI for bilateral fluid collections, diffuse atrophy, evidence of head injury. If suspected and no other history available, drug/toxin screen.

DIFFERENTIAL DIAGNOSIS: From the EEG perspective, alcoholism and closed head trauma are the frequent pathological causes. It rarely occurs postictally and with hydrocephalus.

PROGNOSIS: Little dependable literature on significance of this finding. Significance depends on clinical context (e.g., postictal states can suppress voltage). By itself, it has no prognostic significance.

Clinical Electrophysiology. By © Peter W. Kaplan and Thien Nguyen.
Published 2011 Blackwell Publishing Ltd.

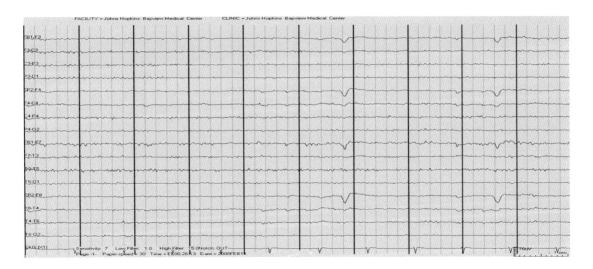

This EEG shows a low-voltage fast beta pattern. There is no posterior or diffuse alpha, theta, or delta activity. Ensure that the EEG recording has the usual interelectrode distances as decreased distance lowers recorded voltage and can produce a similar pattern. Ensure that arousal stimuli have been applied and that eye closure was noted. This pattern is seen in 6–7% of the normal adult population. Alpha/background activity voltage diminishes with age, partly due to increased skull thickness and bone. Posttraumatic patients with this pattern are occasionally deeply obtunded.

REFERENCE:

1. Maulsby RL and Kellaway P . *The Normative Electroencephalographic Data Reference Library*. Final report. NAS 9–1200. Washington, DC: National Aeronautics Space Administration 1968.

8. Alpha coma

CICU, MICU, NICU, SICU, ER

After cardiorespiratory arrest, head trauma.

CLINICAL CORRELATION: By definition, the patient has to be in coma. The patient is eyes closed, but her or she may open to stimuli. Arms posture or withdraw to pain; brainstem reflexes—pupil reactions, vestibulo-ocular reflex, gag, spontaneous breathing—are often present in alpha coma.

ETIOLOGY: It is most frequently reported after CRA (10–23%) [1], less frequently after infection, metabolic dysfunction, head trauma, drugs (e.g., carbamazepine), seizures, stroke, heat stroke, and hypoxia. Cardiorespiratory arrest, infection, metabolic dysfunction, head trauma, seizures, stroke, hypoxia, and drugs.

CLINICAL EVALUATION: Examine for brainstem reflexes and assess Glasgow coma scale. Look for evidence of rare toxic or metabolic causes if CRA is not known.

ANCILLARY TESTING: CT/MRI might show laminar necrosis. Consider Complete metabolic pane and toxin screen, and somatosensory evoked potential (SSEP) for prognosis.

DIFFERENTIAL DIAGNOSIS: In paralyzed patients, ensure that the patient is not awake. Tip-off is lack of EEG reactivity to stimuli, anterior distribution of alpha activity, and if the patient is not paralyzed, presence of eye blink artifact. Alpha frequency patterns (AFPs) can be seen in the locked-in syndrome, but are usually reactive and over the posterior head region. The patient is awake. It rarely occurs with an apallic syndrome. There is a slight resemblance to REM sleep patterns. Posterior AFPs can occur in Grade 1 postanoxic coma (posterior, reactive) with good prognosis [1].

PROGNOSIS: After anoxia/CRA or stroke, the prognosis is almost universally poor; meta-analysis indicates 88 and 90% mortality, respectively. After hypoxia without cardiac arrest 61% mortality; after drugs only 8%. If the EEG shows reactivity, most patients awaken, but few have a meaningful recovery [2]. Almost all patients without EEG reactivity die [1, 2].

Consider SSEPs for further prognosis-—if the N20 is absent, then the outcome is death or persistent vegetative state [1]. Interpret with caution after anesthetics or early (<24 hours) in the clinical course.

TREATMENT: No effective treatment. The EEG pattern evolves into other patterns. The effect of hypothermia is unknown.

Clinical Electrophysiology. By © Peter W. Kaplan and Thien Nguyen. Published 2011 Blackwell Publishing Ltd.

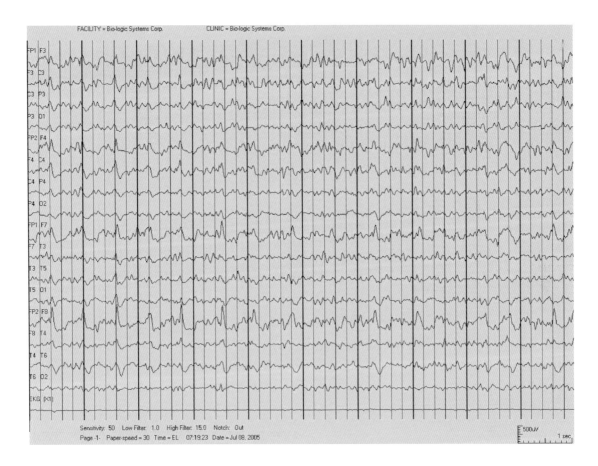

This EEG shows generalized AFP [3] but also some higher frequency beta activity. There is also anterior rhythmic activity with sharp waves. This EEG segment has used a high-frequency filter of 15 Hz to minimize artifact in the illustration.

In alpha coma, the alpha frequencies appear diffusely, but may be more prominent anteriorly. The record usually shows no reactivity to stimuli. AFP may be transient and evolve from a burst-suppression pattern or other pattern, or to another pattern, as in this case. Similar patterns may include slower frequencies in the fast theta range [4] but with similar implications.

REFERENCES:

1. Berkhoff M, Donati F, Bassetti C. Postanoxic alpha (theta) coma: A reappraisal of its prognostic significance. *Clin Neurophysiol* 2000;111:297–304.

2. Kaplan PW, Genoud D, Ho TW, Jallon P. Etiology, neurologic correlations and prognosis in alpha coma. *Clin Neurophysiol* 1999;110:205–213.

3. Westmoreland BF, Klass, DW, Sharbrough FW, Reagan TJ. Alpha coma. Electroencephalograpic, clinical, pathologic and etiologic correlations. *Arch Neurol* 1979;32:713–718.

4. Young GB, Blume WT, Campbell VM, Demelo JD, Leung LS, McKeown MJ, McLachlan RS, Ramsay DA, Schieven JR. Alpha, theta and alpha-theta coma: A clinical outcome study utilizing serial recordings. *Electroencephalogr Clin Neurophysiol* 1994;91:93–99.

9. Spindle coma [1–5]

SICU, CICU, MICU

Seen with head trauma, cardiac arrest, seizures, stroke, and drugs.

CLINICAL CORRELATION: By definition, the patient has to be in coma. Eyes closed but may open to stimuli. Arms posture or withdraw to pain; brainstem reflexes—pupil reactions, vestibulo-ocular reflex, gag, spontaneous breathing—usually present in patients with spindle coma.

ETIOLOGY: It is most frequently reported after head injury; midbrain and brainstem strokes; encephalopathy, hypoxia, drugs, and seizures.

EVALUATION: Examine brainstem reflexes and assess Glasgow coma scale.

ANCILLARY TESTING: MRI may reveal pontomesencephalic pathology. Otherwise test for drug or toxicology screen. For prognosis after CRA, suggest somatosensory evoked potentials (SSEPs).

DIFFERENTIAL DIAGNOSIS: In paralyzed patients, ensure that the patient is not asleep. When due to drug causes, or if seen postictally, patients may be hypersomnolent or still experiencing sedative medications that induce sleep.

PROGNOSIS: Overall mortality is 23%. There is a poor prognosis after cerebrovascular accidents (72% mortality); better after hypoxia (38%), CRA (20%), trauma (15%), drugs/seizures (0–10%) mortality. All patients with reactive spindle coma survived [1]. Spindle coma is rare in children and about a third recovers without deficits—causes include head trauma, drowning, encephalitis, seizures and drugs. Consider SSEPs for further prognostication if caused by CRA. If the cortical SSEP N20 is absent in an anoxic-ischemic etiology, then the predictable outcome is death or persistent vegetative state [3]. Interpret with caution after anesthetics or early (<24 hours) in the clinical course. See also the section on SSEPs.

TREATMENT: No specific treatment. This EEG pattern may evolve to other patterns. The effect of hypothermia on the significance of this finding is unknown. Some physicians have used methylphenidate to induce arousal, but this is viewed as controversial.

Clinical Electrophysiology. By © Peter W. Kaplan and Thien Nguyen. Published 2011 Blackwell Publishing Ltd.

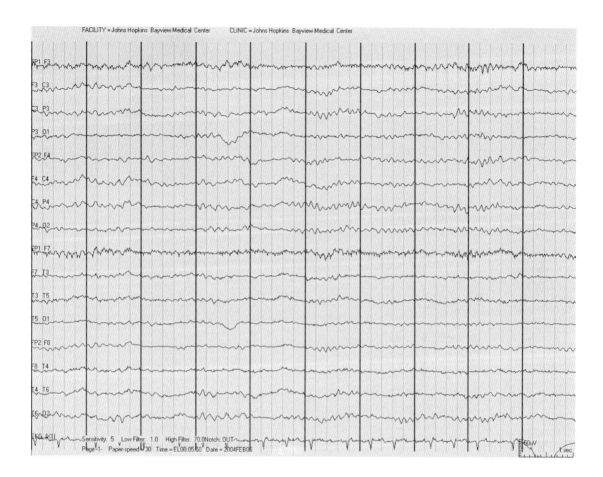

This EEG shows bursts of frontocentral 10-Hz spindles on a delta background. The pattern may be reactive or unreactive to stimuli. It may be a transient pattern, which evolves to a waking alpha or other pattern.

REFERENCES:

1. Britt CW. Nontraumatic "spindle coma". Clinical EEG and prognostic features. *Neurology* 1981;31:393–397.

2. Chatrian G-E, White LE. Sleep EEG patterns in certain comatose states after injuries in the head. *Electroencephalogr Clin Neurophysiol* 1963;15:272–280.

3. Hansotia P, Gottschalk P, Green P, Zais D. Spindle coma: Incidence, clinicopathological correlates and prognostic value. *Neurology* 1981;31:83–87.

4. Kaplan PW, Genoud D, Ho TW, Jallon P. Etiology, neurologic correlations and prognosis in early spindle coma. *Clin Neurophysiol* 2000;111:584–590.

5. Horton EJ, Goldie WD, Baram TZ. Rhythmic coma in children. *J Child Neurol* 1990;5:242–247.

10. Low-voltage suppressed pattern

CICU, MICU, NICU, SICU

Usually after cardio-respiratory arrest may occur with anesthesia [1–4].

CLINICAL CORRELATION: When an EEG shows minimal activity, the patient shows no movements, reaction to pain, or other clinical cortical responses. GCS = 3. Brainstem reflexes may be present.

ETIOLOGY: Usually it occurs after cardiac arrest and less frequently anoxia, high-dose central nervous system suppressant drugs; however, EEG usually shows some bursts of higher voltage activity during a 20-minute recording.

CLINICAL EVALUATION: The need to establish cause of coma is paramount. Ascertain any history before coma onset; exclude anesthetic, barbiturate, or drug effect.

ANCILLARY TESTING: CT, MRI, organ failure, tox screen for cause of coma.

Somatosensory evoked potentials/cortical potentials if absent, indicate zero prognosis for return of consciousness. After CRA, MRI might show laminar necrosis.

DIFFERENTIAL DIAGNOSIS: Rarely the pattern occurs in patients with high doses of cortical suppressants (barbiturates, benzodiazepines, propofol); however, the EEG then usually shows some bursts of higher voltage activity during a 20-minute recording.

Technical problems may cause a flat EEG: check the biological calibration and recording/display sensitivity.

PROGNOSIS: After anoxia/CRA head trauma or stroke prognosis is zero for return to consciousness (check calibration, recording parameters for "electrocerebral inactivity" and for suppressant drugs). In rare cases patients may persist in a vegetative state.

TREATMENT: No effective treatment. Pattern has terminal significance. The effect of hypothermia on the prognostic significance of this pattern is not clear.

Clinical Electrophysiology. By © Peter W. Kaplan and Thien Nguyen.
Published 2011 Blackwell Publishing Ltd.

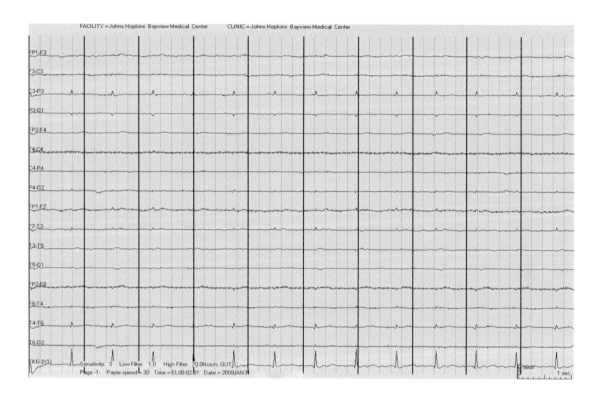

This EEG shows generalized suppression with no cortical activity above 2 μV. There are residual muscle and ECG artifacts. The tracing shows no reactivity to noxious stimuli. Ascertain that no technical cause for absent cortical activity is present. This pattern may have evolved from a burst-suppression, alpha coma, or other pattern. The presence of this pattern is not synonymous with brain death (which is a clinical diagnosis). EEG reports may reflect "electrocerebral inactivity" (if performed correctly to include core temperature above 35°C, absence of anesthetic drugs, use of double-interelectrode distance, testing of each electrode's impedance and presence, minimum 30-minute recording, and appropriate high- and low-frequency filtering).

REFERENCES:

1. Bassetti C, Scollo-Lavizzarri G. Prognostic value of EEG in post-anoxic coma after cardiac arrest. *Eur Neurol* 1987;26:161–170.
2. Pagni CA, Courjon J. Electroencephalographic modifications induced by moderate and deep hypothermia in man. *Acta Neurochir* 1964;13:35–49.
3. Synek VM. Prognostically important EEG coma patterns in diffuse anoxic and traumatic encephalopathies in adults. *J Clin Neurophysiol* 1988;2:161–174.
4. Wijdicks EFM, Hijdra A, Young GB, Bassetti CL, Wiebe S. Practice parameter: prediction of outcome in comatose survivors after cardiopulmonary resuscitation (an evidence-based review): Report of the quality standards subcommittee of the American Academy of Neurology. *Neurology* 2006;67:203–210.

11. Burst/suppression

CICU, MICU, SICU, NICU

Seen after CRA, with anesthesia or during the management of status epilepticus [1–5].

CLINICAL CORRELATE: Eyes closed, but may open congruent with the EEG bursts of epileptiform activity; patients may have facial or limb myoclonus; eyelid twitching, vertical nystagmus; chewing movements and tonic posturing. Caveat for general neurological/brainstem examination: corneal reflexes and eye opening may be difficult to determine because eye opening may be due to epileptic bursts of activity. In the context of coma, this pattern indicates an overwhelming, diffuse cerebral insult [1].

ETIOLOGY: This EEG pattern is seen after CRA, hypothermia, and intoxication with CNS suppressants (e.g., barbiturate overdose) [1–5]; end-stage CNS disease.

CLINICAL EVALUATION: Examine brainstem reflexes and assess Glasgow coma scale. The physical examination is often compromised by the patient's movement, which is caused by the epileptic activity.

ANCILLARY TESTING: Review causes of CNS suppression—toxin screen; history of anoxia/CRA.

Consider CT/MRI for evidence of laminar necrosis, herniation, or other massive CNS insult. For prognosis after CRA, somatosensory evoked potentials (SSEPs).

DIFFERENTIAL DIAGNOSIS: The EEG during anesthesia, treatment with propofol, midazolam, or barbiturates can produce these patterns.

PROGNOSIS: After anoxia/CRA, prognosis is almost universally poor—no better than persistent vegetative state (PVS) [5]. If the pattern persists after 48 hours in the absence of sedatives or hypothermia, no patients return to consciousness. The effect of hypothermia is unclear, and itself may induce this pattern. Consider testing with SSEPs for further prognostic help. If the N20 is absent, then the outcome is death or PVS. Interpret bust suppression with caution after anesthetics or early (<24 hours) in the clinical course. It is rarely seen with pachygyria, Ohtahara's syndrome, and early myoclonic encephalopathy when bursts typically last 2–6 seconds, and suppression periods last 2–10 seconds.

TREATMENT: After CRA, no palliative effect. In our experience, no return to consciousness after CRA whatever the management.

Clinical Electrophysiology. By © Peter W. Kaplan and Thien Nguyen.
Published 2011 Blackwell Publishing Ltd.

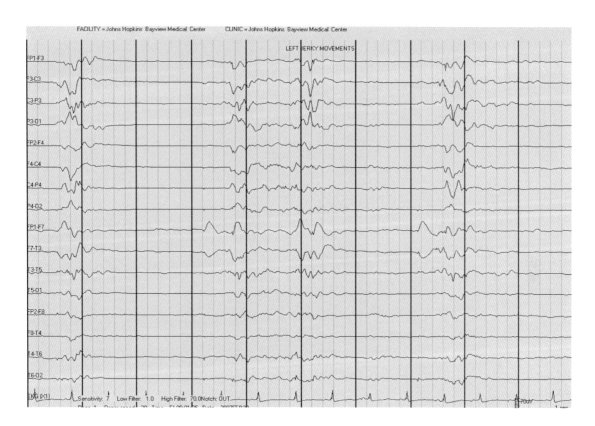

This EEG shows generalized bursts of polymorphic epileptiform discharges lasting from less than a second to several seconds, interspersed with periods of suppression (activity <20 μV) usually lasting 2–10 seconds, but they can be longer [1].

REFERENCES:

1. Prior PF. *The EEG in Acute Cerebral Anoxia.* Assessment of cerebral function and prognosis in patients resuscitated after cardio-respiratory arrest. Amsterdam: Excerpta Medica 1973;314.
2. Haider I, Matthew H, Oswald I. Electroencephalographic changes in acute drug poisoning. *Electroencephalogr Clin Neurophysiol* 1971;30:23–31.
3. Pagni CA, Courjon J. Electroencephalographic modifications induced by moderate and deep hypothermia in man. *Acta Neurochir* 1964;13:35–49.
4. Synek VM. Prognostically important EEG coma patterns in diffuse anoxic and traumatic encephalopathies in adults. *J Clin Neurophysiol* 1988;2:161–174.
5. Wijdicks EFM, Hijdra A, Young GB, Bassetti CL, Wiebe S. Practice parameter: prediction of outcome in comatose survivors after cardiopulmonary resuscitation (an evidence-based review): Report of the quality standards subcommittee of the American Academy of Neurology. *Neurology* 2006;67:203–210.

12. Diffuse slowing—toxic encephalopathy—baclofen [1–6]

MICU, WARD, ER

Seen with toxins, for example, baclofen, cefepime, and ifosfamide. EEG pattern can also be seen with metabolic problems, liver and renal insufficiency.

CLINICAL CORRELATES: Depending on the severity of drug toxicity, patients may complain of sedation, nausea, vomiting, vertigo, or depression. Some patients, particularly the elderly, may be drowsy and confused to the point of stupor. The eyes may be open or closed, and may open to stimuli. The patient can usually speak. Confusion, flapping tremor, and myoclonus may dominate the picture. In lighter coma, the patient can follow commands, localize to pain, and have intact brainstem reflexes. In deeper coma from baclofen, the patient may require vasomotor and ventilator support. There may be generalized seizures.

ETIOLOGY: The principal impairment is that due to central nervous system toxicity. In the case given here, baclofen, a γ-amino butyric acid (GABA) analog which binds to bicuculline-insensitive GABA-B receptors in the brainstem, is the most commonly used drug for spinal cord spasticity. Baclofen may be therapeutic at lower doses, but toxic at higher oral or intrathecal doses.

CLINICAL EVALUATION: Standard general neurological examination, with particular attention to myoclonus, seizures, and the need for cardiovascular and ventilatory support.

ANCILLARY TESTING: Look for electrolyte abnormalities, other causes of toxicity—high ammonia level, an abnormal liver profile, a positive toxin screen, other neuroleptic drugs. Test specifically for particular drugs.

DIFFERENTIAL DIAGNOSIS: *Clinical*—Toxic encephalopathies may cause confusion and sedation, but several (lithium, baclofen, tricyclic antidepressants, ifosfamide, and some antibiotics) may also induce tremors, myoclonus, and seizures. Lithium may be suspected by the clinical signs of cerebellar, basal ganglia, and peripheral nerve dysfunction.

EEG—Similar EEG pictures can be produced by cephalosporins and bismuth. Classical triphasic waves (TWs) (e.g., with hepatic or even renal failure) are blunter and usually of lower frequency than the discharges of nonconvulsive status epilepticus (NCSE). TWs may increase (rarely decrease) with arousal. Background activity can be present with either TWs or NCSE. TWs resolve with benzodiazepines, but the patient fails to improve. Fifty-nine percent of patients with TWs may have nonmetabolic encephalopathies [2].

PROGNOSIS: This largely depends on the degree of drug toxicity and the concurrent organ failure that accompanies it (acute renal failure). Baclofen, cefepime, and ifosfamide toxicities are largely reversible.

TREATMENT: The cornerstone is supportive ICU care and treatment of organ failure. If NCSE is suspected as a differential diagnosis, then a trial of lorazepam 2–4 mg may improve NCSE clinically and either on EEG; benzodiazepines may worsen encephalopathies.

Clinical Electrophysiology. By © Peter W. Kaplan and Thien Nguyen.
Published 2011 Blackwell Publishing Ltd.

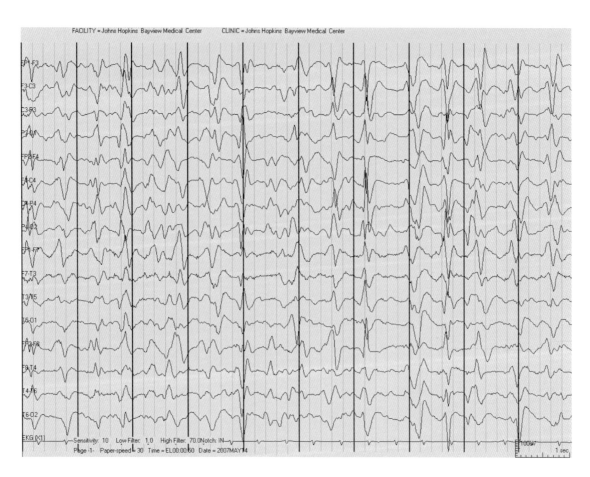

This EEG shows a mixture of diffuse, slower frequencies in the theta and delta range, as well as generalized triphasic waves (see also triphasic waves). Cases of baclofen toxicity have shown increased slow activity, decreased fast frequencies, periodic activity, TWs, semiperiodic epileptiform discharges, generalized epileptiform, and burst-suppression patterns. TWs are often dominant anteriorly, with an anteroposterior lag on a referential montage. Toxic and metabolic causes of diffuse slowing and TWs cannot be clearly distinguished on EEG.

REFERENCES:

1. Abarbanel J, Herishanu Y, Frisher S. Encephalopathy associated with baclofen. *Ann Neurol* 1985;17:617–618.

2. Sundaram MB, Blume WT. Triphasic waves: Clinical correlates and morphology. *Can J Neurol Sci* 1987;14: 136–140.

3. Bahamon-Dussan JE, Celesia GG, Grigg-Damberger MM. Prognostic significance of EEG triphasic waves in patients with altered state of consciousness. *J Clin Neurophysiol* 1989;6:313–319.

4. Blume WT. Drug effects on EEG. *J Clin Neurophysiol* 2006;23:306–311.

5. Fakhoury T, Abou-Khalil B, Blumenkopf B. EEG changes in intrathecal baclofen overdose: A case report and review of the literature. *Electroencephalogr Clin Neurophysiol* 1998;107:339–342.

6. Boutte C, Vercueil L, Durand M, Vincent F, Alvarez JC. EEG contribution to the diagnosis of baclofen overdose. *Clin Neurophysiol* 2006;36:85–89.

13. Diffuse slowing—metabolic encephalopathy—lithium [1–6]

MICU, WARD, ER

CLINICAL CORRELATES: Depending on the severity of lithium toxicity, patients have variable degrees of lethargy, but often exhibit evidence of cortical (slowing or even dementia), corticospinal (spasticity), extrapyramidal (rigidity and tremor), cerebellar (ataxia), and peripheral nerve impairment. Myoclonus and seizures frequently occur with significant toxicity. The eyes may be open or closed, and may open to stimuli. The patient is confused and may be able to speak. Confusion, rigidity, and myoclonus may dominate the picture. In lighter coma, the patient can follow commands and localize to pain; brainstem reflexes present.

ETIOLOGY: The principal CNS impairment is that due to lithium toxicity, but concurrent metabolic problems (acute renal failure), intercurrent infection and fever complicate the picture and contribute to long-term morbidity.

CLINICAL EVALUATION: Examine for evidence of neurological deficits in the broad spectrum of CNS/peripheral nervous system-affected systems. This will include evaluation of the level of consciousness, cognitive function, nystagmus, tone (rigidity and spasticity), limb coordination (tremor and ataxia), and reflexes. Recent infection or dehydration is frequent precipitants of lithium toxicity.

ANCILLARY TESTING: Look for electrolyte abnormalities, other causes of toxicity—ammonia level, liver profile, toxin screen, other neuroleptic drugs. Obtain an MRI for white matter disease. The clinical state may persist after normalization of the lithium level and lag as lithium levels are being corrected.

DIFFERENTIAL DIAGNOSIS: On EEG, triphasic waves (TWs) are blunter and usually of lower frequency than the discharges of nonconvulsive status epilepticus (NCSE). TWs may increase (rarely decrease) with arousal. Background activity can be present with either TWs or NCSE. TWs resolve with BZPs, but the patient fails to improve. Fifty-nine percent of patients with TWs may have non-metabolic encephalopathies [2].

PROGNOSIS: This largely depends on the degree of lithium toxicity and the concurrent organ failure that accompanies it (acute renal failure). Mortality and prolonged morbidity with ICU support over several weeks to months are not rare.

TREATMENT: For lithium toxicity, supportive ICU care and treatment of organ failure determine outcome. There may be a need to treat associated myoclonus and seizures with benzodiazepines and AEDs—consider levetiracetam. If NCSE is suspected as a differential diagnosis, then a trial of lorazepam 2–4 mg may improve NCSE clinically and either on EEG; benzodiazepines may worsen encephalopathies.

Clinical Electrophysiology. By © Peter W. Kaplan and Thien Nguyen.
Published 2011 Blackwell Publishing Ltd.

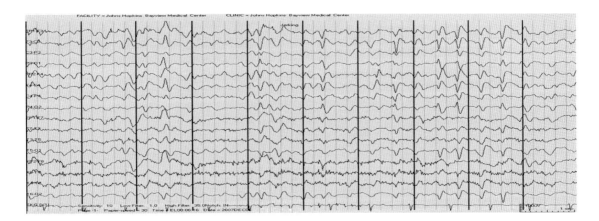

This EEG shows a mixture of diffuse, slower frequencies in the theta and delta range, as well as generalized triphasic waves (see also triphasic waves). TWs are often dominant anteriorly, with an anteroposterior lag on a referential montage. Toxic and metabolic causes of diffuse slowing and TWs cannot be clearly distinguished on EEG.

REFERENCES:

1. Smith SJM, Kocen RS. A Creutzfeldt-Jacob like syndrome due to lithium toxicity. *J Neurol Neurosurg Psychiatry* 1988;51:120–123.

2. Sundaram MB, Blume WT. Triphasic waves: Clinical correlates and morphology. *Can J Neurol Sci* 1987;14:136–140.

3. Bahamon-Dussan JE, Celesia GG, Grigg-Damberger MM. Prognostic significance of EEG triphasic waves in patients with altered state of consciousness. *J Clin Neurophysiol* 1989;6:313–319.

4. Young GB, Bolton CF, Archibald YM, Austin TW, Wells GA. The EEG in sepsis-associated encephalography. *J Clin Neurophysiol* 1992;9:145–152.

5. Blume WT. Drug effects on EEG. *J Clin Neurophysiol* 2006;23:306–311.

6. Kaplan PW, Birbeck G. Lithium-induced confusional states: Nonconvulsive status epilepticus or triphasic encephalopathy? *Epilepsia* 2006;47:2071–2074.

14. Diffuse slowing—metabolic encephalopathy—hypoglycemia [1–3]

MICU, WARD, ER

CLINICAL CORRELATES: Depending on the severity of hypoglycemia, patients have variable degrees of confusion, lethargy, merging into coma. Seizures occur with severe hypoglycemia. In lighter coma, the patient can follow commands, localize to pain, and even in coma the brainstem reflexes are usually present—Babinski reflexes.

ETIOLOGY: Hypoglycemia. Causes include excess insulin, oral hypoglycemic agents, and patients with liver failure.

CLINICAL EVALUATION: Examine for evidence of insulin injections. A nonlateralizing neurological downward progression is seen with increasing hypoglycemia, ranging from confusion to deep coma with relative preservation of brainstem reflexes, but with Babinski responses. Recent infection or dehydration is frequent precipitants.

ANCILLARY TESTING: Look for electrolyte abnormalities and other causes of encephalopathy (toxic and metabolic). The clinical state may persist after normalization of serum glucose level, and thus lag as hypoglycemia is being corrected. Glucose given intravenously in some coma patients may precipitate thiamine deficiency.

DIFFERENTIAL DIAGNOSIS: *Clinical*—The encephalopathic changes are etiologically nonspecific and diagnosis is usually routine because blood chemistry testing is routine. In hypoglycemia, myoclonus, movement disorders, and rigidity are less frequent than in toxic encephalopathies.

EEG—Low-voltage records and/or slowing are nonspecific and can be seen with other acute CNS insult including hypoxia and after seizures.

PROGNOSIS: This largely depends on the degree and duration of hypoglycemia. Prolonged, severe low glucose can result in mild to moderate permanent diffuse cerebral deficit, vegetative states, or death.

TREATMENT: Glucose infusion and supportive ICU care. There may be a need to treat associated myoclonus and seizures with benzodiazepines and AEDs.

Clinical Electrophysiology. By © Peter W. Kaplan and Thien Nguyen.
Published 2011 Blackwell Publishing Ltd.

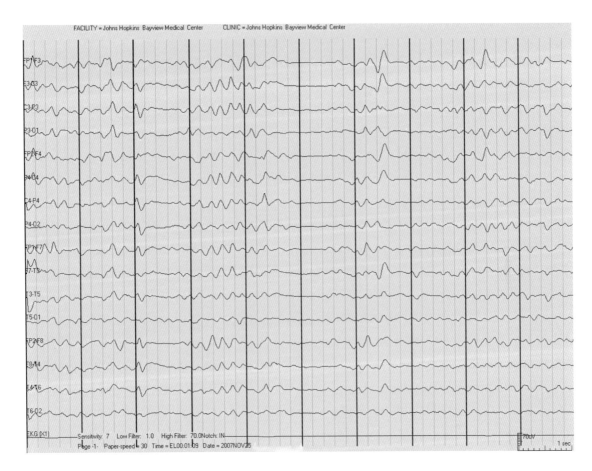

This EEG shows monomorphic 5-Hz theta activity, no posterior waking alpha, and has periods of bilateral suppression. The glucose level was 12 mg/100 mL.

REFERENCES:

1. Lefebre CH, Lefebre B, Skotzek B. An unusual case of insulinoma with confusional states and tonic-clonic seizures diagnosed with the help of long-term video-EEG recording. *Electroencephalogr Clin Neurophysiol* 1990;75:S81 (abstract).
2. Scarpino O, Maurao AM, Del Pesce M. Partial complex seizures and insulinoma: A case report. *Electroencphalogr Clin Neurophysiol* 1985;61:90 (abstract).
3. Prull G, Busch H, Erbsloh F. EEG follow-ups in severe neurological states after hypoglycemia. *Electroencephalogr Clin Neurophysiol* 1970;29:210.

15. Diffuse slowing—limbic encephalopathy [1–6]

CLINICAL CORRELATES: There is a variable clinical presentation with confusion, hallucinations, paroxysmal altered limb and axial tone, hyperoral behavior, and unresponsiveness. There may be catatonia, dyskinesias, short-term memory loss, prominent psychiatric symptoms, a prominent behavioral syndrome with "stickiness" and aggressivity, psychosensory complaints and vegetative complaints, also hypoventilation and autonomic problems.

ETIOLOGY: It was early characterized as a T cell-driven immune response against limbic structures, and has been seen in paraneoplastic or nonparaneoplastic effects of cancers of the lung, breast, thyroid, ovarian teratomas, testicular, and others. Rarely, there is a viral limbic encephalitis or seizures in the limbic structures from various causes.

CLINICAL EVALUATION: General neurological examination looking for abnormalities in tone, hyperoral behavior, and subtle seizures. Look for psychiatric features.

ANCILLARY TESTING: Obtain an enhanced MRI looking for focal abnormalities of the limbic system. Investigate for systemic malignancy with evaluation of lungs, breasts, thyroid and ovaries, body CT, PET (positron emission tomography) scan for tumor localization. Test cerebrospinal fluid for viral, neoplastic, and paraneoplastic antibodies against N-methyl-D-aspartate receptors, voltage-gated potassium channels.

DIFFERENTIAL DIAGNOSIS: *Clinical*—Toxic, metabolic problems (drugs, hyperammonemia, hypocalcemia), celiac disease, Whipple's disease.

Clinical Electrophysiology. By © Peter W. Kaplan and Thien Nguyen.
Published 2011 Blackwell Publishing Ltd.

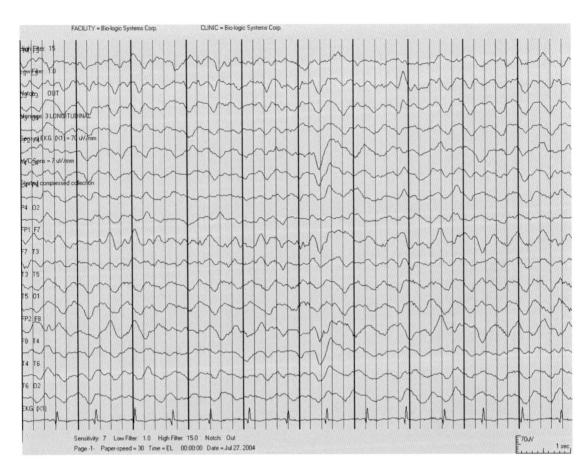

EEG—Toxic and metabolic encephalopathies produce similar patterns.

This EEG shows a medium-voltage waxing and waning theta/delta activity, seeming to shift in frequency over the frontal regions. No epileptiform discharges are evident. The patient was catatonic.

REFERENCES:

1. Brierley JB, Corsellis JAN, Hierons R, Nevin S. Subacute encephalitis of later adult life mainly affecting the limbic areas. *Brain* 1960;83:357–368.
2. Chong JY, Rowland LP, Utiger RD. Hashimoto encephalopathy: Syndrome or myth? *Arch Neurol* 2003;60:164–171.
3. Bataller L, Kleopa KA, Wu GF, Rossi JE, Rosenfeld MR, Dalmau J. Autoimmune limbic encephalitis in 39 patients: Immunophenotypes and outcomes. *J Neurol Neurosurg Psychiatry* 2007;78:381–385.
4. Izuka T, Sakai F, Ide T, Monzen T, Yoshii S, Iigaya, M, Suzuki K, Lynch DR, Suzuki N, Hata T, Dalmau, J. Anti-NMDA receptor encephalitis in Japan. *Neurology* 2008;70:504–511.
5. McKeon A, Marnane M, O'Connell M, Stack JP, Kelly PJ, Lynch T. Potassium channel antibody-associated encephalopathy presenting with a frontotemporal dementia-like syndrome. *Arch Neurol* 2007;64:1528–1530.
6. Graus F, Saiz A. Limbic encephalitis. An expanding concept. *Neurology* 2008;70:500–501.

16. Focal arrhythmic (polymorphic) delta activity

DEFINITION: Slow-frequency (<4 Hz) delta activity without sustained rhythmicity, favoring one hemisphere, often 100- to 150-μV amplitude.

CLINICAL CORRELATES: A patient may have been referred to the electrophysiology laboratory for focal weakness with fluctuating lateralized motor/sensory symptoms. Often, there is focal weakness of the face, arm, and leg; asymmetric reflexes and sensory examination.

ETIOLOGY: This is almost always due to a structural or mass lesion: cerebral infarction, intracranial hemorrhage, abscess, infection, tumor, or focal atrophy. It can rarely occur with ischemia that is not severe enough to cause infarction. It may occur postictally after a focal seizure; this usually resolves rapidly.

CLINICAL EVALUATION: In a general neurological examination, look for cranial nerve, motor or sensory abnormality, evidence of seizures. If there is an abscess, look for an ear or a sinus source of infection.

ANCILLARY TESTING: Obtain imaging to look for structural lesion. Select also MRI sequences sensitive to mild ischemia.

DIFFERENTIAL DIAGNOSIS: On EEG, the significance of focal slowing varies with the clinical context [1–5]. In most patients with structural abnormalities (e.g., an MCA stroke on MRI), there will be continuous, arrhythmic focal delta activity, often with the loss of overlying faster frequencies. With subcortical structural lesions that spare overlying cortex (intra-cranial hemorrhage, abscess), continuous delta may occur with preserved overlying fast activity. This can also be seen with extraaxial compressive meningiomas. When the structural abnormality in the white matter undercuts the cortex (producing arrhythmic delta activity), the concurrent compromise (infarction) of the overlying cortex will also attenuate the focal cortical faster (alpha and beta) frequencies [1–3].

With large focal strokes involving cortical and subcortical areas, the overlying delta activity may be of lower voltage [2]. With large strokes and edema with pressure on midline structures, there may be focal delta with bilateral diffuse delta from midline compromise.

In patients with smaller subcortical lesions, the delta activity may be less persistent or intermittent. Deeply seated lesions may induce more widespread hemispheric or even bihemispheric slowing [4], but often with some preservation of overlying faster activity. Conversely, lacunes even with hemiparesis usually have a normal EEG.

With subclinical ischemia, occasionally insufficient to produce infarction or shortly following a transient ischemic attack, there may be focal delta activity with varying persistence. In some patients, relatively small subcortical strokes will produce intermittent focal delta, but with interspersed periods of relatively normal activity in the same region with preserved, overlying faster (cortical) activity (alpha/beta) frequencies.

In some cases, intermittent phase-reversing focal delta activity with intervening preservation of alpha and beta activities in the same region may represent a more distant epileptic focus, even while a spike or sharp component is absent. In this way, the EEG findings with a particular imaging finding and clinical history may suggest that (a) only a stroke is present; (b) there may be a stroke with a suggestion of seizures; (c) there is subclinical focal ischemia even without frank infarction (critical vascular stenosis); (d) consider a focal structural lesion with mass effect on the midline, and/or herniation; and (e) that there may be postictal slowing, with a relatively minor underlying structural problem.

Clinical Electrophysiology. By © Peter W. Kaplan and Thien Nguyen. Published 2011 Blackwell Publishing Ltd.

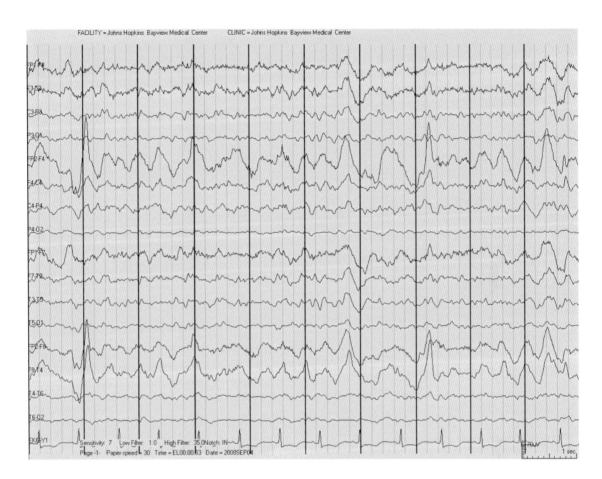

This EEG shows a medium- to high-voltage focal right frontal nonrhythmic (polymorphic) delta activity with preserved faster frequencies, and with little change in EEG pattern on arousal. There are also occasional right frontal sharp waves.

REFERENCES:

1. Gloor P, Kalabay O, Giard N. The electroencephalogram in diffuse encephalopathies: EEG correlates of gray and white matter lesions. *Brain* 1968;91:779–802.

2. Gloor P, Ball G, Schaul N. Brain lesions that produce delta waves on EEG. *Neurology* 1977;27:326–333.

3. Goldensohn ES. Use of the EEG for evaluation of focal intracranial lesions. In: Klass D, Daly D (eds.), *Current Practice of Clinical Electroencephalography*. New York: Raven Press, 1979.

4. Arfel G, Fischgold H. EEG-signs in tumors of the brain. *Electroencephalogr Clin Neurophysiol Suppl* 1961;19:36–50.

5. Bazil CW, Herman ST, Pedley TA. Focal electroencephalographic abnormalities. In: Ebersole JS, Pedley TA (eds.), *Current Practice of Clinical Electroencephalography*, 3rd edn. New York: Lippincott Williams & Wilkins 2003:303–347.

Section B: Periodic patterns of epileptiform discharges or seizures

Periodic discharges (PDs) on the EEG represent a metronomic expression of individual epileptiform discharges. PDs are viewed as being an *irritative* pattern that can be found before or after seizures. They are usually not accompanied by motor signs, and they include PLEDs, BIPLEDs, PLEDs-plus, generalized periodic epileptiform discharge and stimulus-induced rhythmic periodic or ictal discharge. Periodic lateralized epileptiform discharges (PLEDs) are surface-negative discharges with spike, sharp, and polyspike components, with slow-wave complexes. They must be seen on an EEG recording lasting at least 10 minutes. Most patients with PLEDs (83–87%) will have seizures. Patients with bilateral independent synchronous PLEDs (BIPLEDs) also have seizures (78%). With GPEDs, 32–90% may have seizures [1, 2]. Together, these multiple case series [3] show the close relationship between PLEDs and seizures (74–90%), and between PLEDs and status epilepticus (SE) (10–66%). Most patients (94%) had seizures, and therefore PLEDs have been viewed by some as possibly being a "terminal phase of SE." Conversely, others believe that PLEDs per se are not ictal, arguing that their static, nonevolving patterns are an irritative phenomenon and do not represent frank seizure activity [4, 5]. Thus, depending on the situation, PDs can be seen as lying along an ictal–interictal continuum [5, 6].

17. Pseudoperiodic lateralized epileptiform discharges

MICU, CICU, NICU, SICU

Seen in childhood and adults with structural CNS lesions, strokes, tumors, or infections.

Definition

PLEDS: An acute or chronic EEG pattern consisting of discharges with sharp or sharp-and-slow waves; spikes, spike-and-slow waves, or multiple spike-and-slow waves, or complex bursts of multiple spikes with slow waves [3,7–13].

Frequency: PLEDs vary from 3/second to 8/minute [3,7], usually at 1 Hz and last up to 600 ms, vary from 50 to 300 μV. They should be present for at least a 10-minute epoch during a standard EEG recording or be present continuously during a specific behavioral state [9].

CLINICAL CORRELATES: The patient is usually obtunded and may have an asymmetric neurologic examination reflecting the lateralized, structural, cerebral abnormality underlying the PLEDs. Features may wax and wane. Usually, there is a history of recent seizure or change in mental status. There is a close temporal association with seizures—approximately 74–90% [3,7–13]. There may be focal limb movements, head or eye deviation, vocalization, chewing, psychic phenomena including visual or auditory hallucinations, confusion, or autistic behavior [7].

ETIOLOGY: Cerebral infarctions, abscesses, and tumors. Viral and other encephalitides.

CLINICAL EVALUATION: Assess the level of consciousness. Look for lateralized neurological signs, limb movements or twitching, eye deviation. Look for evidence of old stroke or new infection, as well as for sinus or ear source of infection (vesicles of herpes simplex virus (HSV)).

ANCILLARY TESTING: Strokes, abscesses, and tumors can be imaged with head CT. MRI may reveal the early appearance of a viral encephalitis, showing a proclivity for certain brain regions: HSV for frontal and temporal cortex; varicella zoster vasculopathy in white matter and gray–white matter junctions; cytomegalovirus around the lateral ventricles; togavirus encephalitis (e.g., West Nile, Japanese, Eastern and Western Equine encephalitides) around deep-seated white matter, thalami, substantia nigra. Consider cerebrospinal fluid studies for viruses, other infections, but particularly HSV.

DIFFERENTIAL DIAGNOSIS: From the EEG perspective, in partial SE, the discharges are of higher frequency, and clinically, the patient may manifest evidence of an irritative cortical lesion with limb jerks, contraversive head and eye movements, a more clearly defined onset and offset, and with cycling of clinical features. The differentiation between an ictal and an interictal state is largely based on the extent of visible clinical manifestations, the frequency of EEG discharges (usually faster than about 1/second), and the appearance of discrete clinical seizures or an ictal evolution. It is not to be confused with absence status and triphasic waves, which are generalized EEG phenomena.

PROGNOSIS: This depends on the underlying etiology. Usually, PLEDs are transient, lasting from several hours to days or, less commonly, weeks. PLEDs may herald the appearance of a viral encephalitis. PLEDs are often considered to be an "irritative" phenomenon along an "ictal–interictal continuum."

TREATMENT: The use of AEDs may prevent superadded appearance of clinical seizures, but do not address the underlying cerebral disease. Often parenteral benzodiazepines along with a longer-acting AED are tried. More

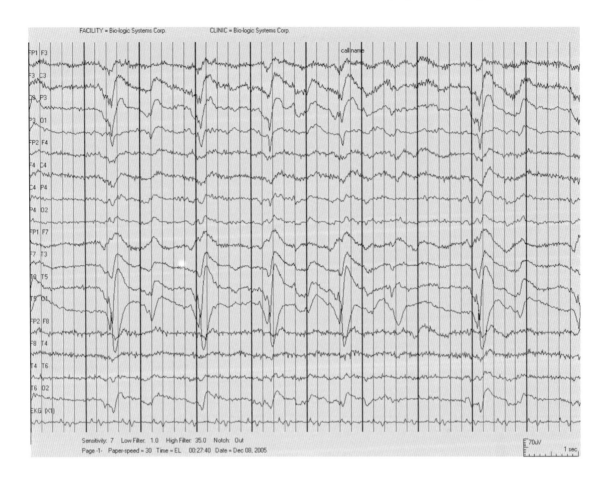

intensive attempts at PLED suppression with higher doses of benzodiazepines or anesthetic agents are unsuccessful, and run up against the tradeoff of iatrogenic problems of hypotension and cardiac dysrhythmia, versus the perceived benefit of seizure suppression. Intensive treatment PLEDs (as opposed to seizures) is controversial.

This EEG shows pseudoperiodic lateralized epileptiform discharges PLEDs at less than 1/second, with some background activity.

REFERENCES:

1. Husain AM, Mebust KA, Radtke RA. Generalized periodic epileptiform discharges: Etiologies, relationship to status epilepticus, and prognosis. *J Clin Neurophysiol* 1999;16:51–58.
2. Yemisci M, Gurer G, Saygi S, Ciger A. Generalized periodic epileptiform discharges: Clinical features, neuroradiological evaluation and prognosis in 37 adult patients. *Seizure* 2003;12:465–472.
3. Snodgrass SM, Tsuburaya K, Ajmone-Marsan C. Clinical significance of periodic lateralized epileptiform discharges: Relationship with status epilepticus. *J Clin Neurophysiol* 1989;6:159–172.
4. Young GB, Goodenough P, Jacono V, Schieven JR. Periodic lateralized epileptiform discharges (PLEDs): Electrographic and clinical features. *Am J EEG Technol* 1988;28:1–13.
5. Pohlmann-Eden B, Hoch DB, Cochius JI, Chiappa KH. Periodic lateralized epileptiform discharges—a critical review. *J Clin Neurophysiol* 1996;13:519–530.
6. Chong DJ, Hirsch. Which EEG patterns warrant treatment in the critically ill? Reviewing the evidence for treatment of periodic epileptiform discharges and related patterns. *J Clin Neurophysiol* 2005;22:79–91.
7. Chatrian GE, Cheng-Mei S, Leffman H. The significance of periodic lateralised epileptiform discharges in EEG: An electrographic, clinical and pathological study. *Electroenceph Clin Neurophysiol* 1964;17:177–193.
8. de la Paz D, Brenner RP. Bilateral independent periodic lateralized epileptiform discharges. *Arch Neurol* 1981;38:713–715.

9. Kuriowa Y, Celesia GG. Clinical sigificance of periodic EEG patterns. *Arch Neurol* 1980;37:15–20.

10. Reiher J, Rivest J, Grand-Maison F, Leduc CP. Periodic lateralized epileptiform discharges with transitional rhythmic discharges: Association with seizures. *Electroenceph Clin Neurophysiol* 1991:78:12–17.

11. Westmoreland BF, Klass DW, Sharbrough FW. Chronic periodic lateralized epileptiform discharges. *Arch Neurol* 1986:43:494–496.

12. Brenner RP. Is it status? *Epilepsia* 2002;43:103–113.

13. Gilden DH. Brain imaging abnormalities in CNS virus infections. *Neurology* 2008;70:84.

18. Bilateral independent pseudoperiodic lateralized epileptiform discharges [1–6]

MICU, CICU, NICU, SICU

DEFINITION: An acute EEG pattern consisting of discharges with sharp or sharp-and-slow waves, spikes, spike-and-slow waves, or multiple spike-and-slow waves, or complex bursts of multiple spikes with slow waves, seen over each hemisphere with different and independent frequency [1–3].

Frequency: It varies from about 1/second to 12/minute, may last up to 600 ms, amplitude up to about 200 μV, but may differ over each hemisphere. Like periodic lateralized epileptiform discharges, they should be present for at least a 10-minute epoch during a standard EEG recording, or be present continuously during a specific behavioral state.

CLINICAL CORRELATES: The patient is usually deeply obtunded; coma in 72%; brainstem reflexes usually present. Rarely, there are limb or facial movements or twitches.

ETIOLOGY: Usually caused by significant multifocal cerebral damage. This occurs typically from encephalitis, anoxia, or multifocal structural disease.

ANCILLARY TESTING: Head CT or MRI to look for structural lesions or evidence of infection. Imaging with CT reveals typical causes such as anoxia (28%), CNS infections (28%), and strokes. It is also seen in epilepsy. It is associated with seizures in more than 60% of patients.

DIFFERENTIAL DIAGNOSIS: In partial SE, the discharges are more frequent and clinically display more "irritative/positive" features of cortical stimulation, that is, limb movement, contraversive head and eye movements. Seizures have a more clearly defined onset, with cycling of clinical features. Differentiation between an ictal and an interictal state is largely based on the degree of visible clinical manifestations, the frequency of EEG discharges (usually faster than about 1/second), and the appearance of discrete seizures or an ictal evolution. Absence status and triphasic waves (TWs) are generalized phenomena but more symmetric. Although TWs may be asymmetric, they do not display a pseudoperiodic pattern. Bilateral independent pseudoperiodic lateralized epileptiform discharges (BIPLEDs) do not typically react to noxious stimuli, while TWs often do.

PROGNOSIS: Poorer prognosis than with PLEDs, largely because the prognosis is determined by the underlying etiology. Usually, BIPLEDs are a transient phenomenon, lasting from several hours to days, or less commonly, weeks. The use of AEDs may prevent superadded appearance of clinical seizures. BIPLEDs (like PLEDs) are often viewed as an "irritative" phenomenon along an "ictal–interictal continuum."

TREATMENT: The patient is often given a trial of parenteral benzodiazepines along with a longer-acting AED. More intensive attempts at BIPLED suppression with more benzodiazepines or anesthetic agents to achieve the benefit of seizure suppression are usually unsuccessful and run up against the tradeoff of iatrogenic hypotension and cardiac dysrhythmia.

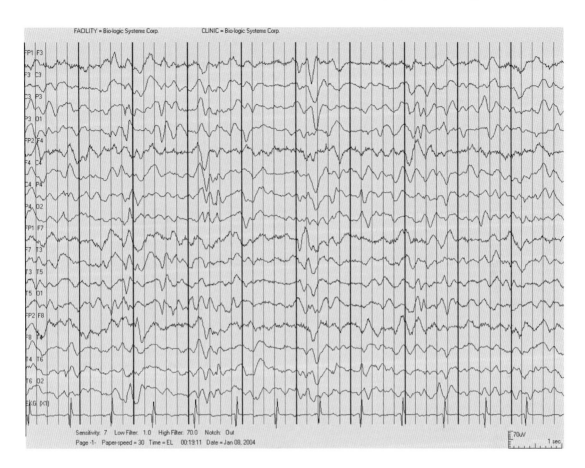

This EEG shows BIPLEDs every 1 to 3 seconds with theta background activity.

REFERENCES:

1. Chatrian GE, Cheng-Mei S, Leffman H. The significance of periodic lateralised epileptiform discharges in EEG: An electrographic, clinical and pathological study. *Electroenceph Clin Neurophysiol* 1964;17:177–193.
2. de la Paz D, Brenner RP. Bilateral independent periodic lateralized epileptiform discharges. *Arch Neurol* 1981;38: 713–715.
3. Kuriowa Y, Celesia GG. Clinical sigificance of periodic EEG patterns. *Arch Neurol* 1980;37:15–20.
4. Snodgrass SM, Tsuburaya K, Ajmone-Marsan C. Clinical significance of periodic lateralized epileptiform discharges: Relationship with status epilepticus. *J Clin Neurolgphysiol* 1989;6:159–172.
5. Westmoreland BF, Klass DW, Sharbrough FW. Chronic periodic lateralized epileptiform discharges. *Arch Neurol* 1986;43:494–496.
6. Husain AM, Megust KA, Radtke RA. Generalized periodic epileptiform discharges: Etiologies, relationship to status epilepticus and prognosis. *J Clin Neurophysiol* 1999;16: 51–58.

19. Generalized periodic epileptiform discharges

MICU, CICU, NICU, SICU, ER

Seen after cardiac arrest, status epilepticus or infection [1–3].

CLINICAL CORRELATES: There are often face or limb myoclonias, eye or eyelid twitching, or vertical nystagmus. Correlation with seizures approximately 90% [2]. Eyes are usually closed, but may open to stimuli. Arms may posture or withdraw to pain; brainstem reflexes—pupil reactions, vestibulo-ocular reflex, gag, spontaneous breathing—present to absent.

ETIOLOGY: In the context of coma, this pattern indicates an overwhelming, diffuse cerebral insult. This pattern is seen after CRA, anoxia, or massive central nervous system (CNS) infection. Generalized periodic epileptiform discharges (GPEDs) may occur as an end-stage of convulsive status epilepticus. It is rarely seen with acute drug toxicity. Rare causes are syphilis and Creutzfeldt-Jakob disease (CJD).

CLINICAL EVALUATION: Examine brainstem reflexes and assess Glasgow coma scale. Look for myoclonias.

ANCILLARY TESTING: Suggest electrolytes, toxin screen for toxic, or metabolic dysfunction. Imaging for infectious causes (e.g., herpes simplex virus or other encephalitides).

DIFFERENTIAL DIAGNOSIS: Epileptiform discharges are sharper and more frequent than triphasic waves or other encephalopathies. The GPED pattern is also consistent with some types of generalized nonconvulsive status epilepticus.

PROGNOSIS: After anoxia/CRA, the prognosis is almost universally poor. If there is background activity above 20 μV, prognosis is better. The effect of hypothermia is unclear. Consider somatosensory evoked potentials (SSEPs) for further prognostication if the cause is CRA. If the cortical N20 is absent on SSEPs, then the outcome is death or persistent vegetative state. Interpret the EEG (and SSEPs) with caution after anesthetics or early (<24 hours) in clinical course.

If there is no anoxia/CRA, then this may represent status epilepticus and the prognosis is better [3]. A trial of antiepileptic drugs is warranted. When etiology is unknown and the pattern does not follow on convulsive status epilepticus, and it is not due to CNS infection or CJD, then the prognosis is guarded and probably poor. Rare exceptions with better prognosis are when it is due to syphilis. With baclofen (where EEG shows background activity and discharges are less frequent), there is a better prognosis for reversibility. The overall mortality in large patient series with toxic, metabolic, infectious, and anoxic causes is approximately 50% [2].

TREATMENT: For seizures, consider a trial of lorazepam 4–8 mg, then phenytoin load; propofol, midazolam, or barbiturates are usually futile. In our experience after CRA, there is no return to consciousness.

Clinical Electrophysiology. By © Peter W. Kaplan and Thien Nguyen.
Published 2011 Blackwell Publishing Ltd.

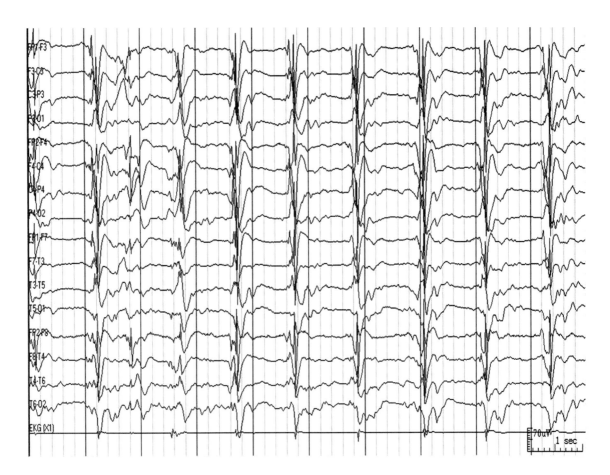

This EEG shows GPEDs without background activity.

GPEDs are generalized epileptiform discharges occupying more than 50% of a 20-minute recording, synchronously and symmetrically over both hemispheres [1]. They occur at short intervals of approximately 0.5–3.0 Hz versus long intervals seen in SSPE.

REFERENCES:

1. Husain AM, Mebust KA, Radtke RA. Generalized periodic epileptiform discharges: Etiologies, relationship to status epilepticus and prognosis. *J Clin Neurophysiol* 1999;16: 51–58.

2. Yemisci M, Gurer G, Saygi S, Ciger A. Generalized periodic epileptiform discharges: Clinical features, neuro-radiological evaluation and prognosis in 37 adult patients. *Seizure* 2003; 12:465–472.

3. Treiman DM, Meyers PD, Walton NY, Collins JF, Colling C, Rowan AJ, Handforth A, Faught E, Calabrese VP, Uthman BM, Ramsay RE, Mamdani MB. A comparison of four treatments for generalized convulsive status epilepticus. Veterans affairs status epilepticus cooperative study group. *N Engl J Med* 1998;339:792–798.

PART 2
Seizures

Section A: The diagnosis of confusional events due to seizures

A consult may be requested for a patient with the sudden onset of poorly described symptoms that involve sensory, motor, autonomic, or limbic features. A patient may describe, for example, perceptions of light flashes, or images; or may describe bizarre clicks, buzzes, sounds, or music; other patients may have just dizziness and vertigo, with nausea and sweating. When these events are brief and stereotyped, the possibility of their being partial seizures arises. With partial seizures, clinical signs and symptoms may simulate a great variety of perceptions or functions, although with a "nonphysiological" quality and evolution. The suspicion of an ictal cause stems from the stereotypy of the events, presence of confusion when present, and often the occurrence of more typical epileptic features such as automatisms or secondary generalization. An account of these typical clinical features of seizures can be found in textbooks on epilepsy and the imitators of epilepsy [1].

With an increased index of suspicion, an EEG may be requested, but the imperfect sensitivity and specificity of EEG should be understood. Also, even epileptiform features on an EEG may be misconstrued, either because they are benign variants or artifacts, or because the particular event under consideration is due to a concurrent problem (e.g., vertigo from inner ear problems in a patient with epilepsy and a "Positive EEG"). The sensitivity of EEG varies for particular seizure or epilepsy types, with the duration of the recording, and whether sleep and wakefulness were both obtained.

Regarding routine 20- to 30-minute outpatient, daytime EEG samples (the "standard" EEG, often without sleep), the pickup rate for true epileptiform abnormalities is 50% or less. For repeated EEGs up to 4, or for prolonged EEGs exceeding an hour, with sleep, the pickup rate rises above 70% for partial seizures and 90% for genetic, idiopathic epilepsies. The gold standard for diagnosis of epileptic events is *epilepsy monitoring* for several days, but the cost–benefit must be weighed for infrequent events. For events occurring several times weekly or more, a few days of monitoring may suffice. For patients who are already in hospital, it is usually easier to embark on *epilepsy monitoring*. This would include patients who are on the general services or in intensive care units. In patients with confusion at the time of the EEG, the test is more sensitive and will often reveal whether a diffuse cortical, diffuse cerebral, focal structural, focal epileptic, or diffuse epileptic process is present. EEGs are good at differentiating psychiatric confusion (normal EEG) from either encephalopathic (different patterns of diffuse abnormality) or epileptic causes.

The simplest ictal problem to diagnose is status epilepticus because the altered clinical state and ictal EEG occur at the same time. That said, there may be lack of consensus on where on an ictal–interictal continuum the patient may lie. See the discussion in the next section for a distillation of these issues. In a nutshell, if seizures are seen on the EEG and the symptoms or signs of interest are present, then status can be diagnosed.

Of similar use is the EEG that shows discrete seizures. There, the diagnosis is as readily made, but the clinical implications differ because of the greater urgency in the need for treatment of status epilepticus. Clusters of frequent convulsive seizures may also pose morbid risk, but the diagnosis is seldom in doubt. Clusters or frequent partial seizures pose intermediate urgency. The therapeutic diseases vary from no antiseizure treatment for discrete reactive seizures (e.g., alcohol, tramadol, or other triggers) to intensive anesthesia for convulsive status epilepticus. Many texts are available for the management of seizures and epilepsy.

The most difficult pickup and lowest yield for EEG is the event for which there is little information from either the patient or bystanders ("Patient found down"), which clinically has resolved days before the EEG and is an isolated incident. In this case, the fishing expedition with EEG is only helpful if the EEG shows paroxysmal abnormalities of sudden phase-reversing delta slowing, or of greater help, epileptiform discharges. In adults, epileptiform discharges rarely occur without a diagnosis of epilepsy (either prior or subsequent); in other words, the false-positive rate is less than 5%.

The section to follow will show different EEG patterns that may occur in patients either confused or with recent confusion. The undifferentiated term "confusion" as an indication for doing an EEG is used to cast a wider net, although clearly more specific histories with "lip-smacking, foaming at the mouth, or head turning with hemi-body jerking" are more likely to yield a helpful EEG (whether it shows epileptiform abnormalities or not). The consultation request may come under a number of forms:

a. As a request for evaluation of a relatively nonspecific symptom, for example, flashes of light, fear, and arm jerking.
b. Because of a history of epilepsy or known seizures that prompt a request for reevaluation.
c. An in-hospital witnessed new event (or event similar to prior ones) suggests a seizure.
d. Ongoing, in-hospital clinical features suggesting status epilepticus.

e. A consultation request stemming from a prior EEG that may have shown epileptiform features.

The EEG figures provided in this section will therefore vary from the isolated temporal lobe spike-slow wave discharge that is highly suggestive of temporal lobe epilepsy, to the diagnostic illustrations of seizures, to figures showing the many types of status epilepticus. In this way the physician can fashion a consultation answer that incorporates the respective significance of the initial clinical question, the need for EEG (or the results therefrom), and the history and examination findings obtained during the consultation. In this way, the significance of either the history or the EEG may be enhanced by the relative specificity of the other. In other words, an EEG showing status epilepticus will trump a nonspecific history of confusion or coma, while a clear temporal lobe EEG spike wave will confirm a history of automatisms, or in another clinical setting, may at least strengthen the suspicion of temporal lobe epilepsy in a patient with poorly described staring episodes.

To best serve this function, the chapter figures begin by demonstrating epileptic discharges over the different brain regions, then in the next section show what seizures may look like over these same regions, and finally end with illustrations of status epilepticus arising from the different brain areas.

20. Frontal lobe simple and complex partial seizures [1–5]

CLINICAL CORRELATES: Frontal lobe seizures are frequently mistaken for psychogenic (nonepileptic) events. Consciousness often is spared, and the manifestations can include emotional, sexual, and delusional content. Supplementary motor area seizures produce uni- or bilateral tonic posturing, a "fencing" posture, or sudden involuntary posturing of an arm or leg causing the patient to reach out for the other limb. The history can be difficult to obtain—auras may consist of bizarre bilateral or unilateral proximal limb or head somatosensory perceptions, numbness, and tingling. When the person has no recollection of subsequent events, then the seizure is *complex partial*. Motor events can include myoclonic jerks. Onset in area 6 can produce vocalization, speech arrest, and palilalia. There may be adversive head movements in almost half of the patients. The patient may experience forced thinking, fear, screaming, complex postural changes, autonomic changes, tonic spasms, or even immobility. Automatisms can consist of movements resembling boxing, cycling, and fishing. There may be drop attacks, grimacing, thrashing, kicking, violent struggling, weeping, laughing, dystonic posturing, and tapping. Dissociative episodes can by inseparable from psychiatric conditions. Events are usually brief (90% <3 minutes and most <30 seconds) and may arouse the patient from sleep.

ETIOLOGY: Any focal structural lesion—cortical dysplasias, hamartomas, gliosis, arteriovenous malformations; idiopathic and familial syndromes.

CLINICAL EVALUATION: Examination is often normal between seizures if the causative lesion is small and nondestructive. Look for lateralized, frontal release signs, lateralized differences in reflexes, or a Babinski sign.

ANCILLARY TESTING: Obtain an enhanced MRI for evidence of focal cerebral lesions such as dysplasias, low-grade astrocytomas, and cavernous angiomas. Positron emission tomography scans can produce a 96% sensitivity and 74% accuracy using quantitative analysis as opposed to 69 and 43%, respectively, with qualitative studies [4].

DIFFERENTIAL DIAGNOSIS: *Clinical*—When the symptoms or manifestations are psychic or sexual, or the patient has dissociations, a psychiatric diagnosis is usually evoked. The movements are occasionally mistaken for movement disorders, or they may be overlooked. Patients may go for years undiagnosed if there is only simple partial or brief complex partial symptomatology. Enquire after events during sleep, blood on the pillow, unexplained accidents. Post-, pre-, or ictal headache may occur.

EEG—Frontal, rhythmic slow activity can be misread for frontal seizures. Further, there may be spread to the temporal areas. Nocturnal frontal epilepsy may have normal interictal studies.

PROGNOSIS: Many patients will remit with anti-epileptic drugs (AEDs) if the underlying cause is not progressive, but a lower proportion than with temporal lobe epilepsy. Management is directed at cause, at suppressing seizures and educating the patient and family on the personal, social, and professional implications of seizures and epilepsy. Just over 50% may become seizure free with extratemporal lesional surgery [5]. Epilepsia partialis continua (a form of frontal motor status) may be largely impervious to medical treatment for months, occasionally responding to subpial transection or resective surgery.

TREATMENT: Consider AEDs for repeated events and imaging to look for a cause. Surgery can be considered for refractory epilepsy.

Clinical Electrophysiology. By © Peter W. Kaplan and Thien Nguyen. Published 2011 Blackwell Publishing Ltd.

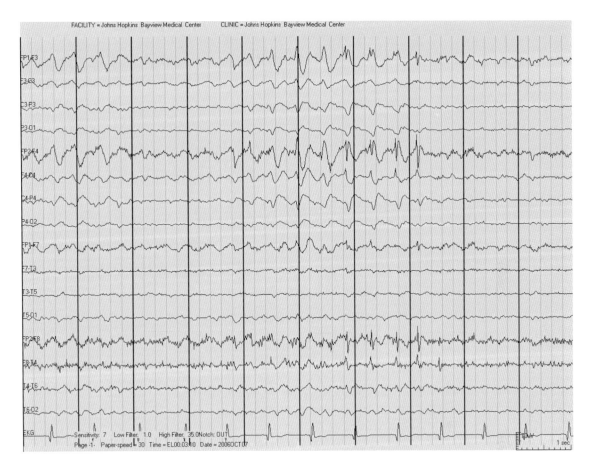

The EEG shows a run of bifrontal epileptiform discharges that are more distinct on the right-hand side.

REFERENCES:

1. Jobst BC, Siegel AM, Thadani VM, Roberts DW, Rhodes HC, Williamson PD. Intractable seizures of frontal lobe origin. *Epilepsia* 2000;41:1139–11452.
2. Williamson PD, Spencer DD, Spencer SS, Novelly RA, Mattson RH.. Complex partial seizures of frontal lobe origin. *Ann Neurol* 1985;18:497–504.
3. Morris HHI, Dinner DS, Luders H, Wyllie E, Kramer R. Supplementary motor seizures: Clinical and electroencephalographic findings. *Neurology* 1988;38:1075–1082.
4. Swartz BE, Khonsari A, Brown C, Mandelkern M, Simpkins F, Krisdakumtorn T. Improved sensitivity of 18-FDG-positron emission tomography scans in frontal and "frontal plus" epilepsy. *Epilepsia* 1995;36:388–395.
5. Talairach J, Bancaud J, Bonis A, Szikla G, Trottier S, Vignal JP, Chauvel P, Munari C, Chodkievicz JP. Surgical therapy for frontal epilepsies. In: Chauvel P, Delgado-Escueta AV, Halgren E, Bancaud J (eds.), *Frontal Lobe Seizures and Epilepsies.* New York, NY: Raven Press 1992;57:707–732.

21. Temporal lobe simple and complex partial seizures [1–5]

CLINICAL CORRELATES: There may be a history of poorly described onset (aura), occasionally with déjà vu, a sense of fear, smell, a rising epigastric sensation, butterflies in the stomach, or dizziness—all representing a simple partial seizure. When the person has no recollection of subsequent events, then the seizure is complex partial (with staring, appearing like he/she is in another world, lip-smacking, lip-licking, or swallowing, fidgety hand movements such as rubbing or picking) or secondarily generalized with head deviation and tonic–clonic movements. Ask for foaming at the mouth, tongue biting and falls. Seizures are usually brief (90% <3 minutes) and may arouse the patient from sleep. There may be a variable degree of confusion, often with a puzzled look. In lateral, neocortical temporal lobe seizures, epigastric auras are rare, and more frequently there are auditory hallucinations, or (with left-sided foci) more prolonged speech impairment. A history should be sought for trauma, central nervous system infection, episodes of staring, accidents, and burns, which suggest earlier instances of seizures.

ETIOLOGY: Any focal structural lesion—infections, trauma, strokes, atrophy, sclerosis, cortical dysplasias, cavernous angiomas, dysembryoplastic neuroepithelial tumors, hamartomas, gliosis, arteriovenous malformations.

CLINICAL EVALUATION: The clinical examination is usually normal. Rare exceptions include the neurocutaneous, genetic syndromes, evidence of trauma, or from symptomatic causes. In older patients, there may be evidence of strokes or mass lesions.

ANCILLARY TESTING: Obtain an enhanced head CT or MRI for evidence of cerebral lesions. In the evaluation for seizure surgery in medically refractory patients, positron emission tomography (PET) and single-photon emission computerized tomography (SPECT) scans may have a place.

DIFFERENTIAL DIAGNOSIS: When the symptoms are those of dizziness and vertigo, presyncope or syncope may be suspected. The movements are rarely mistaken for other conditions—they are usually overlooked. Patients may go for years undiagnosed if there are only simple partial or brief complex partial symptomatology. There is less belief, currently in a temporal lobe "personality." The elderly may have "atypical" episodes with behavioral alterations. Enquire after events during sleep, blood on the pillow, unexplained accidents. Post-, pre-, or ictal headache occurs.

PROGNOSIS: Most patients will remit with antiepileptic drugs (AEDs) if the underlying cause is not progressive. Management is directed at cause, suppressing seizures and education on social/professional implications of seizures. With unilateral refractory foci, temporal lobe surgery can render almost three quarters of selected patients seizure-free.

TREATMENT: AEDs are indicated for repeated unprovoked events (epilepsy). Investigate the underlying causes with MRI as older patients may have strokes, tumors, or infection, while younger patients may have trauma, infection, arteriovenous malformation (AVMs), angiomas, focal atrophy (mesial temporal sclerosis), dysembryoplastic neuroepithelial tumors, and many other causes. For chronic, refractory cases, refer for evaluation of seizure surgery.

Clinical Electrophysiology. By © Peter W. Kaplan and Thien Nguyen. Published 2011 Blackwell Publishing Ltd.

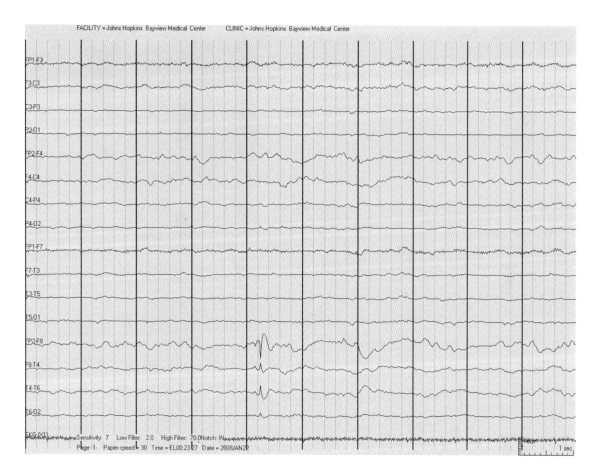

This EEG shows a single spike-slow-wave phase-reversing epileptiform discharge over the right temporal region with concomitant slowing. This helps confirm a diagnosis of temporal lobe seizures. Discharges may increase in sleep.

REFERENCES:

1. Marks WJ, Jr, Laxer KD. Semiology of temporal lobe seizures: Value in lateralizing the seizure focus. *Epilepsia* 1998;39:721–726.

2. Gloor P. Experiential phenomena of temporal lobe epilepsy. Facts and hypotheses. *Brain* 1990;113:1673–1694.

3. Manford M, Fish DR, Shorvon SD. An analysis of clinical seizure patterns and their localizing value in frontal and temporal lobe epilepsies. *Brain* 1996;119:17–40.

4. Mikati M, Holmes G. Temporal lobe epilepsy. In: Wyllie E. (ed.), *In the Treatment of the Epilepsy: Principles and Paractice*, 2nd edn. Baltimore: Williams & Wilkins 1996;401–414.

5. Jackson GD, Berkovic SF, Tress BM, Kalnins RM, Fabinyi GCA, Bladin PF. Hippocampal sclerosis can be reliably detected by magnetic resonance imaging. *Neurology* 1990;40:1869–1875.

22. Parietal lobe simple partial seizures [1–4]

CLINICAL CORRELATES: Typical features are pain in the limbs, face, chest, and rarely in the abdomen. There may be a slow jacksonian sensory march, usually proximally, starting more often in the hand than in the foot, proceeding over seconds up the arm and to the face, headache (simple sensory partial seizures). There is variable loss of consciousness (complex partial seizures). Discomfort may be characterized as "pins and needles," a lack of feeling, "numbness," or perception of altered shape of the limb. Other symptoms include visual illusions and aphasia, vertigo, head and eye deviation, dysmorphic perception of a limb, which include movement and alterations of body image. With spread to motor areas, subtle clonic, myoclonic, or dystonic movements may occur along with gestural automatisms or asymmetric tonic posturing. Negative phenomena such as drop attacks, dysphasia, and paralysis are described.

ETIOLOGY: Any focal structural lesion—infections, trauma, strokes, atrophy, sclerosis, cortical dysplasias, cavernous angiomas, dysembryoplastic neuroepithelial tumors, hamartomas, gliosis, arteriovenous malformations, and porencephalic cysts. One-third of patients have tumors.

CLINICAL EVALUATION: The clinical examination is normal in about half of patients. Look for subtle hyperreflexia, difference in limb and nail size, impairment in two-point discrimination, right–left orientation, visual field defects, and spatial orientation. There may be evidence of neurocutaneous, genetic syndromes, evidence of trauma or of other symptomatic causes. In older patients, there may be evidence of strokes or mass lesions.

ANCILLARY TESTING: Obtain an enhanced head CT or MRI for evidence of cerebral lesions. In the evaluation for seizure surgery in medically refractory patients, positron emission tomography PET and SPECT scans may have a place.

DIFFERENTIAL DIAGNOSIS: *Clinical*—This is an imitator of other painful conditions in that seizures are rarely uniquely or principally painful. Post-, pre-, or ictal headache occurs. Seizures are very rarely the cause for pain at all, but particularly outside the limbs and head. There is usually an identifiable progression, often with secondary generalization and an imageable substrate. Seizure etiology is suggested by the stereotyped, brief progression often with other manifestations of seizures.

EEG—This pattern strongly resembles the mu and alpha frequency physiological patterns, but will extinguish with limb movement or eye opening. Also, it is more arcuate and may resemble wicket spikes.

PROGNOSIS: Partial seizures often respond to antiepileptic drug (AEDs); occasionally the underlying lesion (e.g., malignancy) can cause nonictal and a more refractory pain. Surgery for refractory cases may markedly improve or produce seizure control—75% with tumors and 65% without.

TREATMENT: Consider a trial of AEDs.

Clinical Electrophysiology. By © Peter W. Kaplan and Thien Nguyen. Published 2011 Blackwell Publishing Ltd.

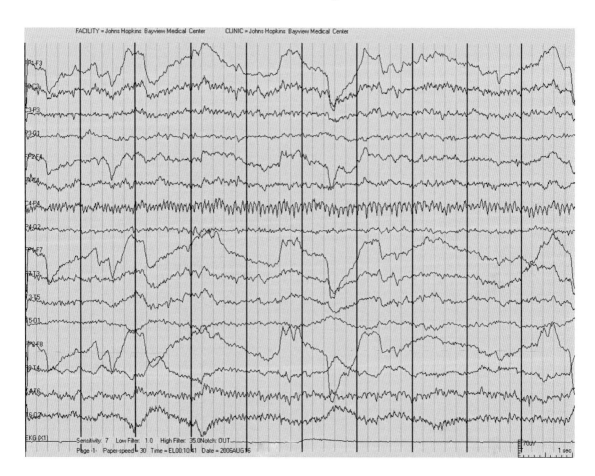

This EEG shows runs of high-frequency sharp waves at more than 10 Hz over the right parietal derivations. Clinical symptoms may occur before or after EEG onset. Background activity is usually present. A high-frequency filter of 35 Hz was used to minimize muscle artifact in this illustration.

REFERENCES:

1. Salanova V, Andermann F, Rasmussen T, Olivier A, Quesney LF. Parietal lobe epilepsy. Clinical manifestations and outcome in 82 patients treated surgically between 1929 and 1988. *Brain* 1995;188:607–627.
2. Williamson PD, Boon FA, Thadani VM, Darcey TM, Spencer DD, Novelly RA, Mattson RH. Parietal lobe epilepsy: Diagnostic considerations and results of surgery. *Ann Neurol* 1992;31:193–201.
3. Seigel AM, Williamson PD, Roberts DW, Thadani VM, Darcey TM. Localized pain associated with seizures originating in the parietal lobe. *Epilepsia* 1999;40:845–855.
4. Cascino GD, Hulihan JF, Sharbrough FW, Kelly PJ. Parietal lobe lesional epilepsy: Electroclinical correlation and operative outcome. *Epilepsia* 1993;34:522–527.

23. Occipital lobe simple partial seizures [1–6]

CLINICAL CORRELATES: The eyes are usually open. The patient may perceive "positive" visual phenomena (one-half to three-fourths of patients). These include dots, flashes, and other simple shapes. These may have color, move and develop into more formed visual images of objects, or brief scenes. Perceived objects may include balls of light, revolving images, and accompanying auditory hallucinations. Transient blindness (40%) or hemifield loss can occur. The patient may be seen to have conjugate eye deviation (adversion) and nystagmus, usually contraversive to the occipital epileptic focus; head deviation to the same side may occur. Seizures in the occipital lobes (representing 5% of symptomatic focal epilepsies) can produce several clinical features. There may be subjective perception of dots, flashes, colored lights, scotomas, amaurosis, hemianopsias, or zig-zags of light (involvement of Brodmann area #17); the patients may note that their eyes/environment are deviating to one side (stimulation of posterior temporoparietal or frontal saccadic regions) [4], often with visual jerking (oscillopsia), eye flutter, or blinking [1–3]. There may be concomitant blinking, dizziness, vertigo, nausea, or headache.

ETIOLOGY: In younger patients, there are genetic focal epilepsies. Symptomatic causes include strokes, trauma, cortical dysplasia, AVMs, cavernous angiomas, and other tumors.

CLINICAL EVALUATION: Examine the visual for field defects (20–60%), although a significant number of patients are unaware of their loss. Look for sudden ictal eye movements, blinking, adversion, and other automatisms.

ANCILLARY TESTING: Obtain MRI for structural cause in the occipital lobe—stroke, mass lesion, or infection. Consider visual field testing.

PROGNOSIS: Many patients respond to antiepileptic drug (AEDs), particularly cryptogenic and stroke patients. There may be seizure freedom in a third to almost half of patients with surgically resected lesional occipital lobe epilepsy.

TREATMENT: AEDs are indicated for repeated seizures. Imaging can reveal an underlying cause (MRI with enhancement).

Clinical Electrophysiology. By © Peter W. Kaplan and Thien Nguyen.
Published 2011 Blackwell Publishing Ltd.

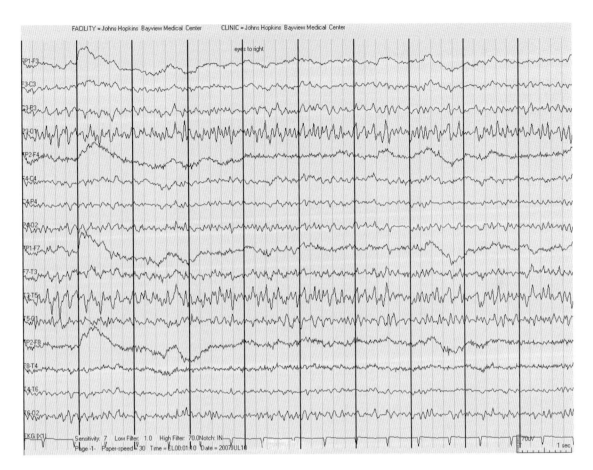

FACILITY = Johns Hopkins Bayview Medical Center   CLINIC = Johns Hopkins Bayview Medical Center

The EEG shows high-frequency polyspike discharges evolving over the left occipital region at 6–16/sec

REFERENCES:

1. Salanova V, Andermann F, Olivier A, Rasmussen, T, Quesney LF Occipital lobe epilepsy: Elecroclinical manifestations, electrocorticographay, cortical stimulation and outcome in 42 patients treated between 1930 and 1991. *Brain* 1992;113: 1655–1680.
2. Williamson PD, Thadani VM, Darcey TM, Spencer DD, Spencer SS, Mattson RH. Occipital lobe epilepsy: Clinical characteristics, seizure spread patterns, and results of surgery. *Ann Neurol* 1992;31:3–13.
3. Tusa RJ. Saccadic eye movements, supranuclear control. *Bull Soc Belge Ophtalmol* 1989;237:67–111.
4. Kaplan PW, Lesser RP. Vertical and horizontal epileptic gaze deviation and nystagmus. *Neurology* 1989;39:1391–1393.
5. Kaplan PW, Tusa RJ. Neurophysiologic and clinical correlations of epileptic nystagmus. *Neurology* 1993;43:2508–2514.
6. Allen IM. A clinical study of tumors involving the occipital lobe. *Brain* 1930;80:194–243.

Section B: **Status epilepticus**

The diagnosis of tonic–clonic (convulsive) status epilepticus (CSE) is usually apparent (and yet there are even case series of aggressively treated pseudo-status epilepticus). Some clinical clues to true status epilepticus (SE) are foaming at the mouth, upgoing toes, and the absence of features suggestive of nonepileptic seizures [1, 2]. Frequently after convulsions, the creatine phosphokinase (CPK) is raised and blood pH is low. Clinical details can be found in standard texts. CSE is a neurological emergency, and management involves intubation and parenteral benzodiazepines (we prefer lorazepam 4–8 mg given under controlled conditions with blood pressure monitoring and ventilation). If seizures persist, an anesthetic agent is often then required, such as propofol, midazolam, or pentobarbital. Along the way, phenytoin is often loaded to prevent recurrence of seizures. The utility of intravenous valproate or levetiracetam is still under study. Most hospitals, intensivists, and neurology departments have their respective preferred practices or protocols, applicable in the inpatient setting.

Nonconvulsive status (NCSE) is harder to diagnose and can supervene under a number of guises [3]. Although subtle myoclonus, gaze deviation, catalepsy, and psychiatric features are some of the variety of presentations, the most common ones are eyes-open mutism with facial and limb twitching. The clinical setting also provides a clue. In the emergency room (ER) it may be gaze deviation, myoclonus, and mutism; in psychiatric settings, catatonia, mutism, or psychiatric regression; in patients with mental retardation, it may be "regression of behavioral milestones" and misbehavior. Common forms are focal frontal, bifrontal, or temporal in patients with structural abnormalities or prior epilepsy; generalized forms (on EEG) can occur with neuroleptics, benzodiazepine abuse, and withdrawal, along with an intercurrent infection [4]. Some generalized forms (on EEG) have spread from a unilateral frontal focus.

NCSE overall has a lower morbidity than CSE with mortalities around 3% in patients with known epilepsy and low antiepileptic drug (AED) levels. In ICU/organ failure associated with NCSE (in coma), mortality rises pari passu with the general patient condition [5]. Treatment is therefore less imperative and may often stop short of anesthetic agents, but often warrants use of benzodiazepines. The various case vignettes given will provide the spectrum of clinical and therapeutic issues. Particular approaches to the various types of SE are best sought in relevant reviews and texts.

24. Complex partial status epilepticus—frontal [6–10]

CLINICAL CORRELATES: Consciousness is often preserved. There may be staring and mastication movements with tongue protrusion; hypermotor automatisms; waxing and waning attention; inattentiveness, perseveration, and aphasia. Psychiatric symptoms include hallucinations, delirium, paranoia, and depression. Posterior frontal foci may produce inhibitory motor seizures that can simulate a transient ischemic attack.

ETIOLOGY: It can be any focal structural lesion—typically strokes, trauma, known epilepsy, infections.

CLINICAL EVALUATION: The patient's eyes are usually open, along with psychiatric or behavioral manifestations, or conversely with bifrontal NCSE, obtunded or in coma, occasionally with eye deviation and nystagmus.

ANCILLARY TESTING: Obtain enhanced MRI for evidence of focal cerebral lesions such as strokes, infection, or tumors.

DIFFERENTIAL DIAGNOSIS: *Clinical*—When the symptoms or manifestations are psychic or sexual, or the patient has dissociations, a primary psychiatric diagnosis is usually incorrectly invoked. The movements are occasionally mistaken for movement disorders or they may be overlooked.

EEG—Frontal, rhythmic slow activity can be misread for frontal seizures. Further, there may be spread to the temporal areas.

PROGNOSIS: De novo frontal lobe status in any awake patient may remit with doses of an AED. In comatose patients, comorbid conditions are frequent and patients are usually older; hence, the prognosis is poorer with morbidity in at least 25% of patients. *Epilepsia partialis continua* (a form of frontal motor status) may be largely impervious to medical treatment for months, occasionally responding to subpial transection or resective surgery. See also "Frontal lobe simple and complex partial seizures."

TREATMENT: Benzodiazepines and other parenteral AEDs. Phenytoin, valproate, or levetiracetam has been used. Anesthetic agents are usually avoided in the awake patient. Parenteral benzodiazepines, phenytoin, valproate, levetiracetam, and then anesthetic agents are usually considered in unconscious ICU patients on a case-by-case basis.

Clinical Electrophysiology. By © Peter W. Kaplan and Thien Nguyen.
Published 2011 Blackwell Publishing Ltd.

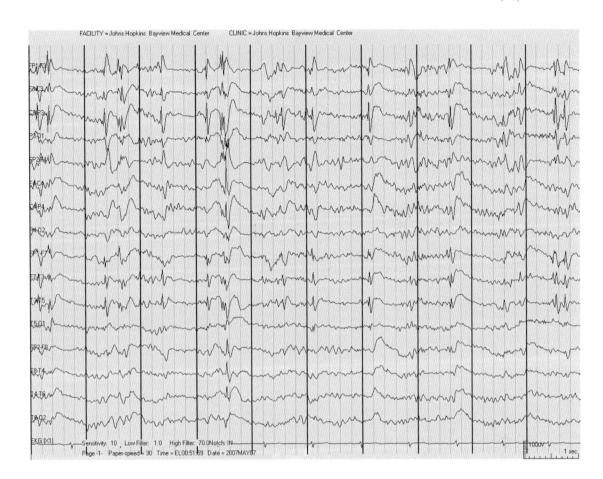

The EEG shows the left frontal spike and poly-spike-slow waves in a mildly confused patient.

REFERENCES:

1. LaFrance WC, Jr, Benbadis SR. Avoiding the costs of unrecognized psychological nonepileptic seizures. *Neurology* 2006;66:1620–1621.

2. *Nonconvulsive status epilepticus*. PW Kaplan, FW Drislane (Eds). Demos Publications. New York, 2009.

3. Kaplan PW. Behavioral manifestations of nonconvulsive status epilepticus. *Epilepsy Behav* 2002;3:122–139.

4. Thomas P, Beaumanoir A, Genton P, Dolisi C, Chatel M. "De Novo" absence status of late onset: Report of 11 cases. *Neurology* 1992;42:104–110.

5. Schneker BF, Fountain NB. Assessment of acute morbidity and mortality in nonconvulsive status epilepticus. *Neurology* 2003;62:1066–1073.

6. Thomas P, Zifkin B, Migneco O, Lebrun C, Darcourt J, Andermann F Nonconvulsive status epilepticus of frontal origin. *Neurology* 1999;52: 1174–1183.

7. Lim J, Yagnik P, Schraeder P, Wheeler S. Ictal catatonia as a manifestation of nonconvulsive status epilepticus. *J Neurol Neurosurg Psychiatry* 1986;49:833–836.

8. Rohr-Le Floch J, Gauthier G, Beaumanoir A. Confusional states of epileptic origin. Value of emergency EEG. *Rev Neurol* 1988;144:425–436.

9. Lee H, Lerner A. Transient inhibitory seizures mimicking crescendo TIAs. *Neurology* 1990;40:165–166.

10. Kaplan PW. Focal seizures resembling transient ischemic attacks due to sub-clinical ischemia. *Cerebrovasc Dis* 1993;3:241–243.

25. Complex partial status epilepticus—temporal [1–4]

CLINICAL CORRELATES: The eyes may be open or closed and may open to stimuli. The patient is confused, disoriented, but usually conversant and may follow commands. The level of consciousness ranges from fully awake with subjective cloudiness to coma. The patient usually localizes to pain; brainstem reflexes intact. Typically in noncomatose patients, there is eyes-open mutism, subtle facial and limb myoclonus, and often catalepsy. Features suggestive of complex partial status epilepticus (CPSE) versus generalized nonconvulsive status epilepticus (GNSE) are complaints of a dreamy state, fear, bizarre smells, déjà vu, autonomic complaints such as sweating, piloerection, tachycardia, evidence of aphasia (versus mutism). There may be staring, lip-smacking, lip-licking, or swallowing, fidgety hand movements such as rubbing or picking, or secondarily generalized with head deviation and tonic–clonic movements. Patients may have prolonged confusional psychiatric and other behavioral abnormalities. More obtunded patients may be lethargic, with contralateral decreased movement; limb automatisms; eye deviation with or without nystagmus.

ETIOLOGY: Any focal structural lesion—infections, trauma, strokes, atrophy. It is common in patients with known temporal lobe epilepsy with poor compliance or low antiepileptic drug (AED) levels.

CLINICAL EVALUATION: The clinical examination will show evidence of confusion, lapses in attention, motor automatisms in eyes-open ambulatory patients. In lethargic or comatose patients in the ICU, there may be subtle movements of the limbs or eyes. Test for neck stiffness. Pay particular attention to the history of cerebral structural abnormality (stroke, trauma, abscess), epilepsy, medication non-compliance, and intercurrent urinary or respiratory infection.

Clinical Electrophysiology. By © Peter W. Kaplan and Thien Nguyen. Published 2011 Blackwell Publishing Ltd.

ANCILLARY TESTING: Obtain an enhanced head CT or MRI for the evidence of cerebral lesions. Prolonged EEG monitoring may be needed in refractory status epilepticus. In de novo patients, consider drugs, encephalitis, and strokes with intercurrent medications and infections (urinary tract infection or pneumonia).

DIFFERENTIAL DIAGNOSIS: Other causes of obtundation with lateralized neurological features, for example, old strokes with encephalopathy. Psychogenic unresponsiveness is not rare. Look for side-to-side head or eye movements, pelvic thrusting, alternating motor limb components.

EEG—Triphasic waves (TWs) are blunter, usually of lower frequency and generalized. Periodic lateralized epileptiform discharges (PLEDs) are of lower frequency, rarely with automatisms, myoclonus, eye or contraversive head deviation. CPSE usually resolves with BZPs, but PLEDs are resistant to regression and the patient rarely improves during treatment.

PROGNOSIS: Prognosis is almost always good when temporal lobe status epilepticus (TLSE) occurs in known epilepsy patients with low AED levels. Prognosis is also good in mildly obtunded patients without multiorgan problems. Very rarely TLSE produces lasting cognitive deficits. In comatose ICU patients, 25–50% of patients have significant morbidity or death.

TREATMENT: Trial of lorazepam 2–4 mg followed by supplementation of the AED the patient may be on. Look for EEG and clinical improvement. Ensure that there is respiratory coverage/support in protected environment for IV BZPs. Phenytoin, valproate, or levetiracetam has been used. Anesthetic agents are usually avoided in the awake patients. Parenteral benzodiazepines, phenytoin, valproate, levetiracetam, and then anesthetic agents are considered in unconscious ICU patients on a

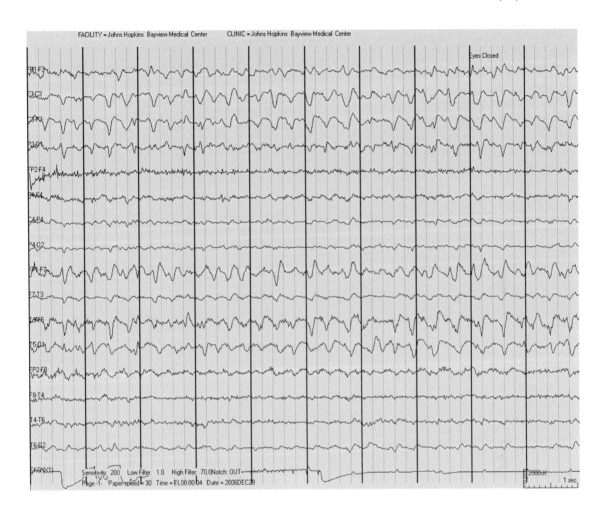

case-by-case basis. This treatment may require prolonged EEG monitoring.

This EEG shows focal epileptiform discharges over the left temporal region at 2–3 Hz, minimally affected by noxious stimuli or arousal. Often there is multifrequency background activity over uninvolved scalp areas, except when the patient is in coma.

REFERENCES:

1. Williamson PD. Complex partial status epilepticus. In: Engel JJ, Pedley TA (eds.), *Epilepsy: A Comprehensive Textbook*. Philadelphia, PA: Lippincott-Raven Publishers 1997;681–699.

2. Young GB, Chandarana PC, Blume WT, McLachlan RS, Munoz DG, Girvin JP. Mesial temporal lobe seizures presenting as anxiety disorders. *J Neuropsychiatry Clin Neurosci* 1995;7:352–357.

3. Fish DR. Psychic seizures. In: Engel JJ, Pedley TA (eds.), *Epilepsy: A Comprehensive Textbook*. Philadelphia, PA: Lippincott-Raven Publishers 1997;543–548.

4. Kirshner HS, Hughes T, Fakhoury T, Abou-Khalil B. Aphasia secondary to partial status epilepticus of the basal temporal language area. *Neurology* 1995;45:1616–1618.

26. Simple partial status epilepticus—parietal [1–3]

CLINICAL CORRELATES: Repeated or continuous proximal tingling or burning sensations. Seizures start more often in the hand than in the foot and proceed over seconds up the arm and to the face. There may be a variable impairment of consciousness (secondary generalization). Discomfort may be "pins and needles," lack of feeling, "numbness," or perception of altered shape of the limb. Pain may occur in other regions, for example, the face, chest, or rarely the abdomen. With spread to motor areas, subtle myoclonic or dystonic movements may occur. See also "Parietal lobe simple partial seizures."

ETIOLOGY: Any focal structural lesion—infections, trauma, strokes, atrophy, sclerosis, cortical dysplasias, cavernous angiomas, dysembryoplastic neuroepithelial tumors, gliosis, arteriovenous malformations, and porencephalic cysts. One-third have tumors.

CLINICAL EVALUATION: The clinical examination is normal in about half of patients. Look for subtle hyperreflexia, difference in limb and nail size, impairment in two-point descrimination, right–left orientation, visual field defects, and spatial orientation. There may be evidence of neurocutaneous, genetic syndromes, evidence of trauma or from symptomatic causes. In older patients, there may be evidence of strokes or mass lesions. In obtunded patients in the ICU in whom the EEG shows seizure activity over the parietal area, the condition is not clearly distinguishable from spread, or overlap from frontal or temporal foci.

ANCILLARY TESTING: Obtain an enhanced head CT or MRI for the evidence of cerebral lesions. In the evaluation for seizure surgery in medically refractory patients, positron emission tomography (PET) and SPECT scans may have a place.

DIFFERENTIAL DIAGNOSIS: *Clinical*—This is a rare imitator of other conditions in that seizures are rarely uniquely or principally painful. Post-, pre-, or ictal headache occurs. Seizures or status epilepticus is very rarely the cause for pain at all, but particularly outside the limbs and head. Seizure etiology is suggested by the stereotyped, brief progression often with other manifestations of seizures.

EEG—This pattern strongly resembles the mu and alpha frequency physiological patterns, but will extinguish with limb movement or eye opening. Also, it is more arcuate and may resemble wicket spikes.

PROGNOSIS: Status epilepticus often responds to antiepileptic drugs (AEDs); occasionally the underlying lesion (e.g., malignancy) can cause nonictal, more refractory pain. Surgery for refractory cases may markedly improve or produce seizure control—75% with tumors and 65% without.

PROGNOSIS: In awake patients, prognosis is good. Seizures or status often responds to AEDs; occasionally the underlying lesion (e.g., malignancy) can cause nonictal, more refractory pain.

TREATMENT: In simple partial status, consider oral use of AEDs—benzodiazepines, or other rapid onset oral AEDs. Look for EEG and clinical improvement. Ensure that there is respiratory coverage/support in protected environment for intravenous benzodiazepines. Anesthetic agents are usually avoided in the awake patient. Parenteral benzodiazepines, phenytoin, valproate, levetiracetam, and then anesthetic agents can be considered in unconscious ICU patients on a case-by-case basis. This treatment may require prolonged EEG monitoring.

Clinical Electrophysiology. By © Peter W. Kaplan and Thien Nguyen. Published 2011 Blackwell Publishing Ltd.

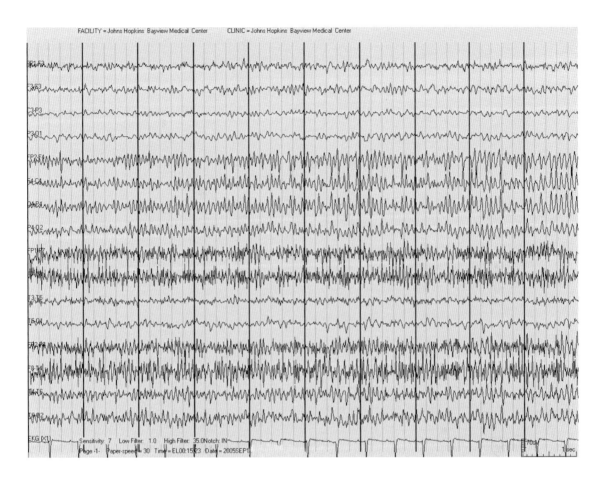

This EEG shows runs of high-frequency sharp waves more than 12 Hz over the right parietal area. There is muscle artifact obscuring both frontal regions. The use of a high-frequency filter set at 35 Hz helped differentiate muscle artifact above 20 Hz from polyspikes over the parietal region at 10–15 Hz.

REFERENCES:

1. Matthews R, Franceschi D, Xia W, Cabahug C, Schuman G, Bernstein R, Peyster R. Parietal lobe epileptic focus identified on SPECT-MRI fusion imaging in a case of epilepsia partialis continua. *Clin Nucl Med* 2006;31:826–828.
2. Feinberg TE, Roane DM, Cohen J. Partial status epilepticus associated with asomatognosia and alien hand-like behaviors. *Arch Neurol* 1998;55:1574–1576.
3. Hopp J, Krumholz A. Parietal lobe status epilepticus. In: Kaplan PW, Drislane F (eds.), *Nonconvulsive Status Epilepticus*. New York: Demos Publications, in press.

27. Simple partial status epilepticus—occipital [1–4]

CLINICAL CORRELATES: The eyes may be open or closed. The eyes often conjugately deviate away from the seizure focus along with nystagmus in the same direction. Rarely, gaze is ipsiversive. Occipital epileptic activity may be continuous or exist as multiple seizures with return to baseline and eyes to midline between seizures. Patients may be aware of the seizure and describe the perception of movement, jumping, or visual hallucinations. There may be amaurosis. Patients may be confused and conversant; others may be more obtunded. The level of consciousness ranges from fully awake with visual symptoms to coma. Alternately, the patient may be unresponsive with head and eye deviation and epileptic nystagmus away from the temporo-parieto-occipital focus, which is usually at high frequency (>10 Hz) at seizure start, but slows to about 3 Hz when the patient is obtunded, constituting a complex partial seizure. This may be followed by the secondary generalization. Ongoing partial occipital status may occur as multiple isolated but frequent seizures (up to every several minutes) without return to baseline, or as a waxing and waning epileptiform spike or sharp wave complex, continuously, usually at 0.75–1.5 Hz. See also "Occipital lobe simple partial seizures."

ETIOLOGY: Any focal structural lesion—infections, trauma, strokes, atrophy, sclerosis, cortical dysplasias, cavernous angiomas, dysembryoplastic neuroepithelial tumors, gliosis, arteriovenous malformations, and porencephalic cysts. One-third have tumors.

CLINICAL EVALUATION: Evaluate for eye movements. Test for visual field defects. Patients may demonstrate nystagmus, head and eye deviation.

ANCILLARY TESTING: Request a head CT/MRI for temporo-occipital junction structural abnormalities.

DIFFERENTIAL DIAGNOSIS: *Clinical*—Other encephalopathies and TLSE occur only rarely with nystagmus, head, and eye deviation.

EEG—Periodic lateralized epileptiform discharges (PLEDs) are of lower frequency. Occipital, intermittent rhythmic delta activity is blunted and rarely sustained.

PROGNOSIS: Good. In an awake patient, status epilepticus usually responds to antiepileptic drugs (AEDs). In comatose patients, comorbidities and neurologic state dictate a poorer outcome.

TREATMENT: Consider a trial of oral benzodiazepine (BZPs). Others advocate using lorazepam 2 mg (under controlled conditions), followed by supplementation of the AED, if the patient is on an AED. Look for EEG and clinical improvement. Ensure that there is respiratory coverage/support in a protected environment for IV BZPs. Anesthetic agents are usually avoided in the awake patient. Parenteral benzodiazepines, phenytoin, valproate, levetiracetam, and then anesthetic agents are usually considered in unconscious ICU patients on a case-by-case basis. This treatment may require prolonged EEG monitoring.

Clinical Electrophysiology. By © Peter W. Kaplan and Thien Nguyen.
Published 2011 Blackwell Publishing Ltd.

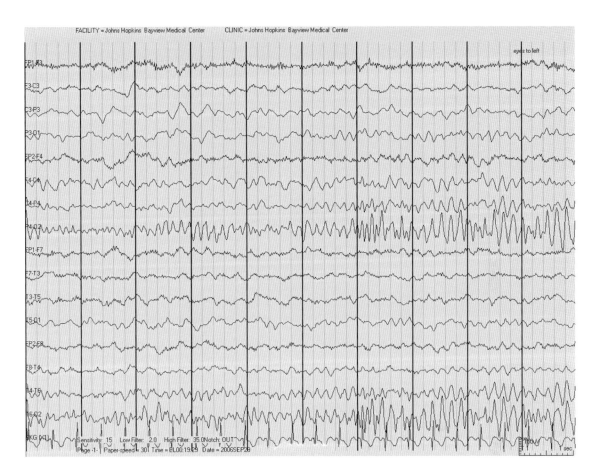

This EEG shows focal epileptiform discharges over the occipital region, initially at 10–12 Hz. There is progressive slowing of the occipital discharge frequency, with an increase in voltage. Eye deviation occurred shortly after ictal onset.

REFERENCES:

1. Sowa MV, Pituck S, Prolonged spontaneous complex visual hallucinations and illusions as ictal phenomena. *Epilepsia* 1989;30:524–526.

2. Sawchuk KS, Chruchill S, Feldman E, Drury I. Status epilepticus amauroticus. *Neurology* 1997;49:1467–1469.

3. Barry E, Sussman NM, Bosley TM, Harner RN. Ictal blindness and status epilepticus amauroticus. *Epilepsia* 1985;26:577–584.

4. Kaplan PW, Tusa RJ. Neurophysiologic and clinical correlations of epileptic nystagmus. *Neurology* 1993;2508–2514.

28. Generalized nonconvulsive status epilepticus [1–9]

CLINICAL CORRELATES: The eyes may be open or closed, or may open to stimuli. The patient is typically confused, disoriented, but usually conversant when he or she present to the ER and may follow simple or even complex commands. The level of consciousness ranges from fully awake, with subjective cloudiness, to coma. In the ICU, the patient is usually lethargic and may have myoclonus and intercurrent tonic–clonic seizures.

ETIOLOGY: In awake or mildly confused patients, concurrent metabolic problems such as hyperammonemia or uremia are not typical. Conversely, there are often infectious problems such as urinary tract infection (URI) or upper respiratory tract infection (URTI), medication burden, cerebral atrophy, and abuse of benzodiazepines. Patients with known generalized epilepsy may have nonconvulsive status epilepticus (NCSE) with low antiepileptic drug (AED) levels. In ICU patients there is usually a combination of strokes, atrophy, toxic, metabolic, or other central nervous system (CNS) insults, and the generalized nonconvulsive status epilepticus (GNSE) may be secondarily generalized on the EEG.

CLINICAL EVALUATION: Perform a global physical and neurological examination, looking for neck stiffness (meningoencephalitis), external evidence of trauma (hemorrhage, contusion). In mildly affected conditions, the patient often localizes to pain and brainstem reflexes are almost always intact. Typically in noncomatose patients, there is eyes-open mutism, subtle facial and limb myoclonus, and often catalepsy.

Pay particular attention to the medication list: look for lithium, recent antibiotics (cefepime), baclofen, benzodiazepines, phenothiazines, recent intercurrent urinary or respiratory infection. In ICU/comatose patients, there may be global decrease in Glasgow coma scale, with or without brainstem reflexes and with localizing or nonlocalizing CNS signs.

DIFFERENTIAL DIAGNOSIS: *Clinical*—Encephalopathies and psychogenic unresponsiveness. Beware of locked-in states, vegetative states, and abulia (see these sections).

EEG—Triphasic waves (TWs) are blunter and usually of lower frequency than discharges of NCSE. TWs may increase (rarely decrease) with arousal, while NCSE epileptiform discharges rarely do. EEG background activity can be present in either TWs or GNSE. TWs resolve with BZPs, but the patient typically fails to improve, while those with NCSE typically improve clinically after IV BZPs.

PROGNOSIS: This largely depends on the underlying cause. Excellent in de novo, reactive causes and in genetic idiopathic generalized epilepsy (IGE) (childhood absence epilepsy (CAE), juvenile myoclinic epilepsy (JME)) when due to low AEDs. Prognosis is less clear in atypical absence status in syndromes such as Lennox–Gastaut syndrome, Landau–Kleffner syndrome, epilepsy with electrical status epilepticus (ESES), or Ring 20 chromosome where the underlying condition is often associated with cognitive impairment or decline. Prognosis is poor when presenting as electrographic status in postanoxic coma or with multiorgan failure. Given the demographic distribution of aged patients, the overall prognosis (all causes excepting ICU/coma patients) is good.

TREATMENT: In lightly affected patients, consider oral benzodiazepines or rapid-acting oral AED. In more affected patients, consider a trial of lorazepam 2–4 mg to look for EEG and clinical improvement. Parenteral agents must be given in a protected environment. In awake patients, IV valproate or levetiracetam has been used. In obtunded patients, further treatment may require EEG monitoring and other AEDs or anesthetic agents, usually in an ICU.

Clinical Electrophysiology. By © Peter W. Kaplan and Thien Nguyen. Published 2011 Blackwell Publishing Ltd.

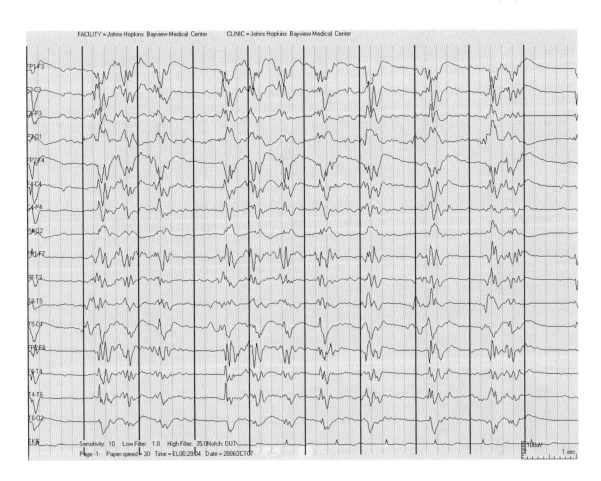

The tracing shows bursts of polyspike-slow waves with suppressed background in a comatose patient after cardiac arrest.

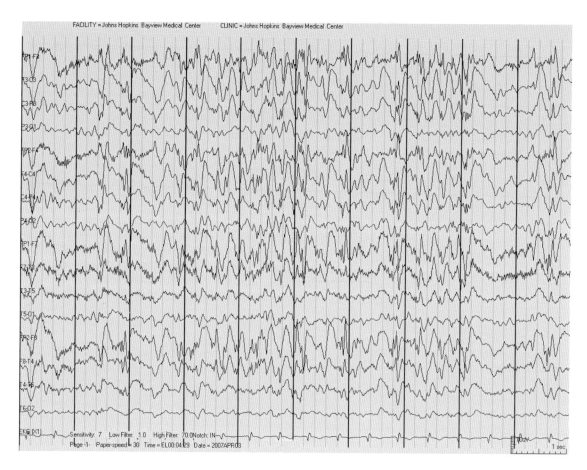

FACILITY = Johns Hopkins Bayview Medical Center   CLINIC = Johns Hopkins Bayview Medical Center

Sensitivity: 7   Low Filter: 1.0   High Filter: 70.0 Notch: IN
Page -1-   Paper-speed = 30   Time = EL00:04:29   Date = 2007APR03

This EEG shows bursts of generalized polyspike-wave discharges with intervening background in a mildly confused patient, several months after a brief cardiac arrest.

REFERENCES:

1. Kaplan PW. Behavioral manifestations of non-convulsive status epilepticus. *Epilepsy Behav* 2002;3:122–139.
2. Agathonikou A, Panayiotopoulos CP, Giannakodimos S, Koutroumanidis M. Typical absence status in adults: Diagnostic and syndromic considerations. *Epilepsia* 1998;39:1265–1276.
3. Baykan B, Gokyigit A, Gurses C, Eraksoy M. Recurrent absence status epilepticus: Clinical and EEG characteristics. *Seizure* 2002;11:310–319.
4. Thomas P, Valton L, Genton P. Absence and myoclonic status epilepticus precipitated by antiepileptic drugs in idiopathic generalized epilepsy. *Brain* 2006;129:1281–1292.
5. Dziewas R, Kellinghaus C, Ludemann P. Nonconvulsion status epilepticus in patients with juvenile myoclonic epilepsy: Types and frequencies. *Seizure* 2002;11:335–339.
6. Drislane FW, Schomer DL. Clinical implications of generalized electrographic status epilepticus. *Epilepsy Res* 1994;19:111–121.
7. Treiman DM. Electroclinical features of status epilepticus. *J Clin Neurophysiol* 1995;12:343–362.
8. Thomas P, Beaumanoir A, Genton P, Dolisi C, Chatel M. "De novo" absence status of late onset: Report of 11 cases. *Neurology* 1992;42:104–110.
9. Kaplan PW. Prognosis in nonconvulsive status epilepticus. *Epileptic Disord* 2000;2:185–193.

PART 3
Conditions of prolonged unresponsiveness

A frequent call for neurological consultation from intensive care units and chronic care centers is for the evaluation of chronically unresponsive patients. The clinical question usually revolves around whether the patient is comatose, vegetative, locked-in, or possibly minimally conscious. Rarely, there may be catatonia—a psychiatric state of inertia. Because the management and prognosis can be markedly different among these diagnoses, an accurate determination is essential. One study has highlighted this problem by finding that many patients diagnosed as being in a vegetative state (VS) were locked-in syndrome (LIS). At the very least it is important to know if the patient is awake, hearing and suffering (LIS), or unconscious (coma or persistent vegetative state). There are some regional, national, or statewide regulations that affect the care or its discontinuation in one or other of these conditions, such as with the minimally conscious state (MCS).

Coma aside, clinical examination will determine and diagnose all states of prolonged unresponsiveness. In some patients, electrophysiology can support one or other possibility, or even exclude other considerations (psychogenic unresponsiveness, nonconvulsive status epilepticus (NCSE)), but electroencephalography (EEG) findings, particularly with persistent vegetative state (PVS), may be quite variable (see PVS case). A printed set of characteristics of these states allows a comparison of the various clinical features. Following are some outlines and considerations in the various states of unresponsiveness.

Section A: Locked-in syndrome, minimally conscious state, vegetative state, and coma: disorders of consciousness and responsiveness

These conditions often present major challenges to the diagnostician when doing neurological consultations. The respective diagnoses usually have markedly different clinical and prognostic implications. A patient with LIS is sentient, can be awake and alert, and can hear and remember what is said. She or he can feel and suffer both mentally and physically. Comatose patients are not known to suffer or remember events during periods of unconsciousness. MCSs lie in between, and less is known about memory and prognosis.

The diagnostic challenge is in the gathering and interpretation of clinical signs at the bedside, and garnering more information than can usually be gathered during a brief consultation. Problems arise because the bedside evaluation of remaining brain function in severely brain-damaged patients often varies from time to time, and can be based on quite limited, elicited patients' reactions. The clinical diagnosis depends on conclusions drawn from reactions to external conditions present during examination. LIS, MCS, and VS are largely clinical diagnoses that may be made without electrophysiological testing. However, there is an increasing amount of data on how such tests may help differentiate wakefulness from coma. There is less information on the differentiation of consciousness from unconsciousness in the awake patient. As many observers have noted, consciousness in not an all-or-none condition.

Table 29.1 summarizes differences among these states.

Table 29.1 Glasgow coma scale[a]

Best motor response	
Obeying commands	6
Localizing to pain	5
Withdrawing to pain	4
Abnormal flexion (decorticate)	3
Extensor response (decerebrate)	2
None	1
Best verbal response[b]	
Oriented	5
Confused conversation	4
Inappropriate words	3
Incomprehensible sounds	2
None	1
Eye opening	
Spontaneous	4
To speech	3
To pain	2
None	1

Adapted from Teasdale and Jennett [2].

[a]The score for the scale is summed across three components and ranges from 3 to 15. A lower score indicates more severe neurological deficits.
[b]Intubated patients cannot be given a score for the verbal component, so their total scores accordingly range from 2 to 10.

29. Clinical definitions of impaired responsiveness [1–11]

Consciousness

Consciousness, an awareness of self and the environment, until recently has been assessed in patients by their ability to follow some commands. It cannot be measured directly by electrophysiological tests, and the evaluation depends on interpretation of clinical findings. The primary components of consciousness are those of arousal and awareness. Arousal is maintained by ascending brainstem connections that project to the thalami and thence to the cortices. Usually, the presence or absence of brainstem reflexes helps to localize the source of unresponsiveness to problems involving the brainstem, or higher up, in the cortex. However, brainstem reflexes can be selectively abolished by focal strokes or trauma, rendering the patient de-efferented. In this state, the patient is awake but not able to produce movement or manifest some brainstem functions. The second component of awareness depends on the extent of cerebral cortical integrity, along with the subcortical connections among cortical regions. Disruption of significant amounts of cortical connectivity results in various degrees of decreased function to the point of producing an MCS, a VS, or coma. Arguably, these represent a continuum of dysfunction, which has been categorized along testable criteria.

Not conscious and not awake: coma

Coma is characterized by the absence of arousal, usually with eyes closed, and without evidence of awareness of self or the surroundings. It is a variable state of eyes-closed unresponsiveness to verbal, auditory, visual, tactile, or other noxious stimuli. The patient may retain brainstem reflexes (particularly after briefer cardiorespira-

Clinical Electrophysiology. By © Peter W. Kaplan and Thien Nguyen. Published 2011 Blackwell Publishing Ltd.

tory arrests (CRAs)) and severe toxic/metabolic problems, or conversely lose these reflexes with the primary brainstem causes of coma. Coma is transient, progressing to wakefulness or death, usually over days.

It contrasts with VS in that stimulation will fail to elicit eye opening or apparent wakefulness, nor will the patient cycle through identifiable periods of sleep and wakefulness. This state must persist for at least an hour, and surviving patients either awaken or gradually evolve to VS over 2–4 weeks. Table 29.1 provides the Glasgow coma scale.

Imaging may reveal common structural causes, involving the brainstem or both cerebral hemispheres, or uncover bihemispheric compressive disease causing brainstem herniation. For the most part, the etiology of coma determines outcome. Structural (stroke, hemorrhage) and irreversible toxic insults carry the worst prognosis; head trauma outcomes may be intermediate, while reversible metabolic issues or seizures often enable complete recovery.

Minimally conscious and awake: minimally conscious states

An MCS, first described in 2002, is a state of severely altered consciousness. There are minimal but definite behavioral manifestations, demonstrating reactions to and awareness of the environment. Such patients may have varying degrees of attention, have purposeful visual tracking, and may communicate. Criteria include having one or more of following simple commands, speech or gestures indicating a *yes* or *no* answer, actions that are reactive to external stimuli, or uttering intelligible words. Distinctions may be difficult because patients with MCS can have a fluctuating examination, and hence have periods in which there is less evidence of response or tracking. More recently, functional magnetic resonance imaging (fMRI) has demonstrated activity in brain areas of minimally conscious patients in patterns similar to those seen in healthy people. These findings are believed to correspond to conscious cognitive processing. Although these patients show overall little clinical evidence of conscious interactive ability, they must show clear evidence of self-awareness or awareness of the environment as demonstrated by following simple commands, *yes* or *no* responses by speech or gestures, intelligible speech, purposeful behavior not due to reflexive responses. Akinetic mutism, which may be due to bihemispheric damage, resembles the MCS, but many authors avoid this term.

Unconscious and awake: vegetative states

In VS, the patient is awake but shows no evidence of awareness of self or the environment. There is cycling of wakefulness and sleep, but without evidence (during wakefulness) of cognitive processing of external stimuli; the patient is awake but not conscious. A *persistent* VS is that which persists for at least 1 month. It does not imply irreversibility. A *permanent* VS is irreversible and usually occurs about 3 months after nontraumatic brain injury, or 12 months after brain trauma. Such prognostications are most robust after anoxic injury, somewhat less so after brain trauma, and even less certain with other nontraumatic causes of unconsciousness.

Conscious and awake: locked-in syndrome

Introduced by Plum and Posner, this state consists of tetraparesis and the inability to speak. It is due to the interruption of corticospinal and corticobulbar pathways. Patients will be able to sustain eye opening, be aphonic and tetraparetic. They have awareness of self and the environment and are able to communicate by the upper eyelid, blinking vertical or lateral eye movements so as to signal *yes/no* answers.

Electrophysiological investigations of deeper levels of impaired responsiveness—diagnosis and prognosis

In patients with unresponsiveness, there is a wide variety of electrophysiological findings.

Coma
EEG – The EEG of coma often correlates with the depth of coma. As the level of consciousness falls, EEG-dominant frequencies slow to theta and delta range. In coma due to medications, there may be particular EEG patterns of faster activity in the beta range (e.g., from barbiturates and benzodiazepines), or conversely bursts of slowing.

Some marked toxic or medication effects can produce a marked suppression of voltage. Drugs or medications excepted, marked suppression or flat-line tracings forebode a poor to no positive prognosis for recovery of consciousness. The EEG findings also often reflect the *etiology* of coma and hence the prognosis. For anoxia with cardiac arrest, minimal or no EEG brain activity indicates no return to consciousness. Somewhat less grim is a pattern of unreactive alpha or theta frequencies that carry a prognosis of less than 15% chance of return to consciousness. Spindle patterns, however, predict overall a better probability of return to consciousness and is the most favorable of the CRA/anoxia patterns. Similar hierarchies of prognosis exist for traumatic coma. Evoked potentials (EPs) also play a role in coma prognosis. Like EEG, their relevance needs to be seen in the light of the coma etiology. Somatosensory evoked potentials (SSEPs) are helpful in predicting outcome after head trauma and CRA/anoxia. When there are no cortical responses after CRA/anoxia (tested >12 hours after coma onset and without hypothermia), one can predict with 100% accuracy that the patient will not regain consciousness. The prognosis is somewhat better with traumatic causes of coma; occasionally some patients with absent potentials regain awareness. The best outcomes are seen with reversible causes of coma. Not surprisingly, SSEPs are usually present (as they are during anesthesia). Short-latency auditory evoked potentials have also value in the prognostication in traumatic coma and CRA, but are less sensitive than SSEPs and are now not often used. Long-latency auditory responses (N70) have been used to differentiate patients who awaken and are conscious versus those who will be vegetative after drowning, but these results have not been widely replicated. Mismatch negativity testing by some investigators has been helpful in predicting a return to consciousness, but more recent studies are less hopeful.

With P300 cortical responses, the vulnerability to ambient or other testing artifacts has led to little use recently, but older data would suggest that their presence is predictive of return or presence of consciousness.

More recent investigation with fMRI and other conditioned imaging modalities indicates that these tests hold greater potential for diagnosis or prognostication. At this moment, these tests are neither bedside nor inexpensive procedures.

Patients typically evolve over hours to days from comatose states. A typical progression would be from coma to alertness, coma to death, or in a minority of patients

Table 29.2 Different behavioral characteristics in states of prolonged unresponsiveness

	LIS(awake)	MCS(awake, minimally conscious)	VS(awake, not conscious)	Coma(not awake, not conscious)
Visual reaction	Blink	Object recognition Visual present	Startle	None
Eye opening	Volitional	Spontaneous	Spontaneous	Variable according to depth
Spontaneous movement	None	Automatic Object manipulation	Reflexive or simple sequences	Posturing
Reaction to pain	Pupil dilation	Localization	Posturing Withdrawal	Posturing
Follows commands	By eye movement/ blinking	Inconsistent but reproducible		
Affective reaction	Yes	Contingent	Random	None
Speech	None	Intelligible words	Random Vocalization	None
Communication	Yes/No No pauses With eye movements	Unreliable Gestural or verbal Yes/No responses	None	None

Adapted from Fins et al. [4].

from coma to VS. In some reports, progression from coma to VS is not accompanied by a change in EEG. In some cases, EEG change will not be reflected in a clinical change.

VS

EEG – For VS, the EEG may range from normal (in a minority of patients) to a pattern of continuous, generalized, polymorphic delta slowing (the majority of patients) unreactive alpha, theta, or spindle coma patterns, reactive theta background or diffuse suppression to the point of being isoelectric, or exhibiting "electrocerebral silence." The authors concluded that EEG was of limited value in VS.

EPs – In some VS patients, auditory EPs were normal, while in many patients, cortical responses were unobtainable on SSEP testing. In other patients, there was prolongation of central conduction time with normal N20 amplitudes. This was thought to reflect selective synaptic delay in thalamic nuclei.

LIS

There may be EEG evidence of wakefulness or sleep activity, and SSEP evidence (on occasion) that there is interruption of ascending sensory stimuli through brainstem or midbrain structures. Such testing does not evaluate consciousness, and both EEG and SSEP may not reliably separate VS from LIS in some patients. Positron emis-

sion tomography (PET) scans may reveal high cerebral metabolic rates in LIS. The different behavioral characteristics can be found in Table 29.2.

"Functional" electrophysiology and functional imaging evaluation of impaired responsiveness

Longer latency "cognitive" evoked potentials obtained by "oddball" auditory stimuli, N70 and P300 potentials, have been used with greater or lesser success in differentiating the conscious patient from the unconscious. Technical problems may impair the ability to demonstrate the presence of such cognitive-processing potentials even in intact persons, and the absence of potentials may also be seen in patients with more diffuse cerebral problems, but who might be conscious. Nonetheless, this area of event-related cognitive processing remains underexplored in the LIS, with VS, MCS, and coma disorders.

As with MCS and VS, functional imaging holds the greater potential for prognostication. Investigations have ranged from studies of brain death with single photon emission computed tomography (SPECT) where cerebral perfusion or metabolism tracers reveal a "hollow skull phenomenon" to a 50–70% fall in gray matter metabolism in traumatic or anoxic coma (predictive of poor outcome), to PET scanning in VS that may

Table 29.3 Prognosis after anoxic coma using five EEG grades (from 408 cases from the literature)

EEG category	Recovery (%)	Survival with permanent neurological damage (%)	Death (%)
Grade 1	79	10	11
Grade 2	51	13	36
Grade 3	26	7	67
Grade 4	0	2	98
Grade 5	0	0	100

Adapted from Scollo-Lavizzari and Bassetti [10]. Permission to be obtained.

be predictive of functional recovery (albeit rarely) to consciousness. fMRI has been used to study responses to language stimuli, with selective activation seen in some patients.

However, even with functional imaging there may be problems as patients cycle through periods of low arousal and sleep and hence produce decreased values on these imaging techniques. Thus, for "activation" scans, EEG monitoring is essential to avoid such physiological "down" periods.

Table 29.4 Determination of the index of global cortical function assessed between 1 and 3 days after anoxic coma onset

	VEPs	SSEPs	Good outcome (%)
Grade 0	Normal	Normal	
Grade 1	Increased peak II latency Peak VII present	Normal N20, P24, and P27 N30 present	60
Grade 2	Increased peak III latency Peak VII absent	Normal N20 and P24 N30 absent	40
Grade 3	Increased peak III latency No subsequent activities	No subsequent activities No cortical activities	15
Grade 4	No reproducible VEPs ERG present	No cortical activities P14 present	0

Adapted from Guérit et al. [9]. Permission to be obtained. SSEP, somatosensory evoked potential; VEP, visual evoked potential.

Prognosis using electrophysiology

Electrophysiology is optimally used in guiding early *diagnostic* investigation, and excluding other differential considerations, including severe encephalopathy, NCSE, or psychogenic issues.

For *prognosis*, EEG can be used early on after an irreversible insult such as ischemia/anoxia from CRA to help predict outcome and the chances for good, poor, or no recovery (Table 29.3). After anoxic coma, EPs also provide reliable prognostication of a poor or negative outcome. Combined with EPs, an index of global cortical function (see Table 29.4) can also be generated to provide a graded prognostication, but frequently the EP testing resources are not available in many hospitals, excepting some academic centers. Imaging techniques are still largely experimental, but may be useful in individual cases.

When patients reach the chronic stages with LIS, VS, PVS, or MCS, electrophysiology does not accrue further prognostic value.

REFERENCES:

1. Kaplan PW. Electrophysiological prognostication and brain injury from cardiac arrest. *Semin Neurol* 2006;26:403–412.
2. Teasdale G, Jennett B. Assessment of coma and impaired consciousness: A practical scale. *Lancet* 1974;2:81–84.
3. Booth CM, Boone RH, Tomlinson G, Detsky AS. Is this patient dead, vegetative, or severely neurologically impaired. *JAMA* 2004;291(7):870–879.
4. Fins JJ, Master MG, Gerber LM, Giacino JT. The minimally conscious state. *Arch Neurol* 2007;64(10):1400–1405.
5. Kampf A, Schmutzhard E, Franz G, Pfausler B, Haring H-P, Ulmer H, Felber S, Golaszewski S, Aichner F. Prediction of recovery from post-traumatic vegetative state with cerebral magnetic-resonance imaging. *Lancet* 1998;351:1763–1767.
6. Multi-Society Task Force on PVS. Medical aspects of the persistent vegetative state (first of two parts). *N Engl J Med* 1994;330:1499–1508.
7. Laureys S, Owen AM, Schiff ND. Brain function in coma, vegetative state, and related disorders. *Lancet Neurol* 2004;3:537–546.
8. Hansotia PL. Persistent vegetative state. *Arch Neurol* 1985;42:1048–1052.
9. Guérit JM, De Tourtchaninoff M, Soveges L, Mahieu P. The prognostic value of three-modality evoked potentials in evoked potentials (TMEPs) in anoxic and traumatic coma. *Neurophysiol Clin* 1993;23:209–226.
10. Scollo-Lavizzari G, Bassetti C. Prognostic value of EEG in post-anoxic coma after cardiac arrest. *Eur Neurol* 1987;26:161–170.
11. Zandbergen EGJ, Hijdra A, Koelman JHTM, Hart AA, Vos PE, Verbeek MM, de Haan RJ; PROPAC Study Group. Prediction of poor outcome within the first three days of post anoxic coma. *Neurology* 2006;66:62–68.

Section B: Prolonged unresponsive states

30. Locked-in syndrome—brainstem hemorrhage [1–4]

NICU, CICU, MICU, SICU

CLINICAL CORRELATES: There is no purposeful limb or trunk reaction, no speech and no mouth or jaw movements. The patient may be in any of several states, ranging from conscious to a clouded sensorium, a minimally conscious, or be comatose along a continuum. The eyes may be open or closed, or may open variably to commands stimuli, or open spontaneously. Movement below the neck may be reflexive.

CLINICAL EVALUATION: Examine the brainstem reflexes, reactivity to stimuli (look for minimal vertical eye movements to commands). The clinical assessment is largely directed at determining if there is meaningful *yes/no* response to external stimuli. This indicates consciousness. Often, more prolonged observation is needed, as families often report "meaningful" responses not seen by nurses and physicians. Assess the patient's score on the Glasgow coma scale (Tables 29.1 and 29.2).

ANCILLARY TESTING: These states often trigger consults and requests for further investigations for consciousness, persistent vegetative state (PVS), locked-in syndrome (LIS), or prognosis. Consider electrolytes, toxin screen, somatosensory evoked potential (SSEP), and CT or MRI depending on the differential diagnosis (see Tables 29.3 and 29.4).

DIFFERENTIAL DIAGNOSIS: Unreactive patients may be mistaken for patients experiencing no conscious perception (Table 29.2). These patients could be aroused from sleep to wakefulness. Functional magnetic resonance imaging (fMRI) may be found to differentiate conscious patients, but clinical examination is still the basis of diagnosing these "similar" states [1,3,4]. Clinically other causes of de-efferentation are severe peripheral nervous

system disease such as with amyotrophic lateral sclerosis (ALS) or other end-stage causes of total peripheral paralysis.

Coma—A clinical state of eyes-closed unresponsiveness from which the patient cannot be aroused (distinction from sleep) without purposeful response to external stimuli. If the cause is unknown, obtain CT/MRI. If uninformative, look for toxic or metabolic causes.

Vegetative state—The patient is awake (eyes open) but unconscious. The diagnosis of the state is clinical; for causes the evaluation is the same as above. The commonest etiologies are post-cardiorespiratory arrest (CRA) and after head trauma, less commonly after hypoglycemia.

Locked-in syndrome—De-efferented state—awake, conscious but minimal evidence of reaction (vertical/horizontal eye movements to questions). Imaging will usually show a stroke in or evidence of trauma to the midbrain/pontine area. Rarely, it occurs as an end-stage of severe, widespread peripheral paralysis (e.g., ALS, myasthenia gravis (MG), and botulism). It occurs rarely in the intensive care unit (ICU) and operating room (OR) in paralyzed patients (vecuronium, pancuronium) who are inadequately sedated or anesthetized.

Catatonia—A state of psychic and motor unresponsiveness. It is characterized by mutism, akinesia, and negativism and may be seen with schizophrenia, post-traumatic stress disorder, bipolar disease, depression, drug abuse, and overdose. It can occur with strokes, metabolic and autoimmune conditions, encephalitis, adverse reactions to medications, and sudden withdrawal from benzodiazepines. It may be caused by decreased central dopaminergic activity from psychiatric, toxic, medical, or unknown origin.

DISCUSSION: fMRI may be found to differentiate conscious patients from vegetative state (VS), but clinical examination is still the basis of diagnosing these "similar" states [1,3,4]. Clinically other causes of de-efferentation are severe peripheral nervous system disease such as

Clinical Electrophysiology. By © Peter W. Kaplan and Thien Nguyen. Published 2011 Blackwell Publishing Ltd.

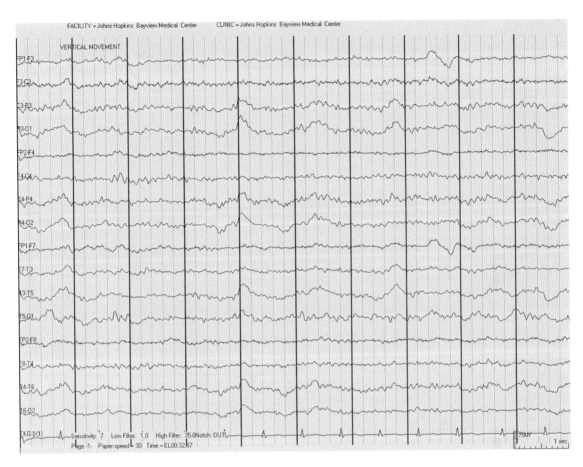

with ALS or other end-stage causes of total peripheral paralysis.

PROGNOSIS: Chronic patients may survive with supportive care, but usually succumb to infection or organ failure. Treatable causes include when it is due to paralyzing agents, which are reversible, and myasthenia gravis so as to reverse limb and speech paralysis. Structural damage to the midbrain and pons and end-stage ALS are irreversible causes of LIS. These conditions are highly distressing to the patient's family, physicians, and nurses, and all may benefit from sensitive and extensive discussions. Consider getting input from an ethics committee.

TREATMENT: Supportive care with chronic ventilation support. All caregivers should be made aware that the patient is sentient, can hear, and experience mental and physical anguish and suffering.

This electroencephalography (EEG) shows 10- to 12-Hz activity superimposed on 0.5- to 1.2-Hz delta frequencies, while the patient is being asked to move her eyes.

In other cases, there may be EEG evidence of wakefulness or sleep activity, and SSEP evidence (on occasion) that there is interruption of ascending sensory stimuli through brainstem or midbrain structures. Such testing does not evaluate consciousness, and both EEG and SSEP may not reliably separate VS from LIS in some patients (see Tables 29.3 and 29.4). PET scans may reveal high cerebral metabolic rates in LIS.

REFERENCES:
1. Cartlidge N. States related to or confused with coma. *J Neurol Neurosurg Psychiatry* 2001;71(Supplement 1): i18–i19.
2. Gutling E, Isenmann S, Wichman W. Electrophysiology in the locked-in-syndrome. *Neurology* 1196;46:1092–1101.
3. Laureys S, Owen AM, Schiff ND. Brain function in coma, vegetative state, and related disorders. *Lancet Neurol* 2004;3:557–546.
4. Young GB. Major syndromes of impaired consciousness. In: Young GB, Ropper AH, Bolton CF (eds.), *Coma and Impaired Consciousness: A Clinical Perspective*. New York: McGraw-Hill 1998:39–78.

31. Vegetative state—postanoxia [1–12]

NICU, CICU, MICU, SICU

CLINICAL CORRELATES: There is no purposeful limb or trunk reaction to outside command. There is neither speech nor language. The eyes may be open, closed, or may open unreliably to sound, stimuli, or open spontaneously. Movement below the neck may be reflexive.

ETIOLOGY: It is most commonly found after cardiac arrest, with the initial presentation being that of coma. It can be seen after severe head trauma; following causes of diffuse intracerebral edema with widespread ischemia from vascular compromise; and more rarely with drowning, carbon monoxide poisoning, hypotension, and/or anoxia during anesthesia. Also, it occurs with severe, diffuse encephalitis, and strokes producing bilateral frontal ischemia.

CLINICAL EVALUATION: Examine the brainstem reflexes and look for reactivity to stimuli (look for minimal vertical eye movements to command seen in locked-in syndrome). The clinical assessment is largely directed at determining if there is meaningful *yes/no* response to external stimuli. This indicates consciousness. Often, more prolonged observation is needed, as families often report "meaningful" responses not seen by nurses and physicians. Assess the patient's score on the Glasgow coma scale.

ANCILLARY TESTING: These states often trigger consults and requests for further investigations for "consciousness," "locked-in syndrome (LIS)," psychogenic unresponsiveness, or prognosis. Consider electrolytes, toxin screen, somatosensory evoked potentials (SSEP), and CT or MRI depending on the differential diagnosis below.

EEG—The EEG may range from normal (in a minority of patients) to a pattern of continuous generalized polymorphic delta slowing (the majority of patients); unreactive alpha, theta, or spindle coma patterns; reactive theta background or diffuse suppression to the point of being isoelectric, or exhibiting "electro-cerebral silence".

EPs—In some vegetative state (VS) patients, auditory evoked potentials (EPs) were normal, while in many patients, cortical responses were unobtainable on SSEP testing. In other patients, there was prolongation of central conduction time with normal N20 amplitudes. This was thought to reflect selective synaptic delay in thalamic nuclei.

DIFFERENTIAL DIAGNOSIS:

Coma—This is a clinical state of eyes-closed unresponsiveness from which the patient cannot be aroused (distinction from sleep) without purposeful response to external stimuli. If the cause is unknown, obtain CT/MRI. If uninformative, look for toxic or metabolic causes.

Locked-in syndrome—LIS is a de-efferented state: the patient is awake, conscious but shows minimal evidence of reaction to external stimuli (vertical/horizontal eye movements to questions). Imaging will usually show a stroke in or evidence of trauma to the midbrain/pontine area. Rarely, it occurs as an end-stage of severe, widespread peripheral paralysis (e.g., amyotrophic lateral sclerosis (ALS), myasthenia gravis (MG), and botulism). It occurs rarely in the ICU and operating room (OR) in paralyzed patients (vecuronium, pancuronium) who are inadequately sedated or anesthetized.

Catatonia—A state of psychic and motor unresponsiveness. It is characterized by mutism, akinesia, and negativism and may be seen with schizophrenia, posttraumatic stress disorder, bipolar disease, depression, drug abuse, and overdose. It can occur with strokes, metabolic

Clinical Electrophysiology. By © Peter W. Kaplan and Thien Nguyen. Published 2011 Blackwell Publishing Ltd.

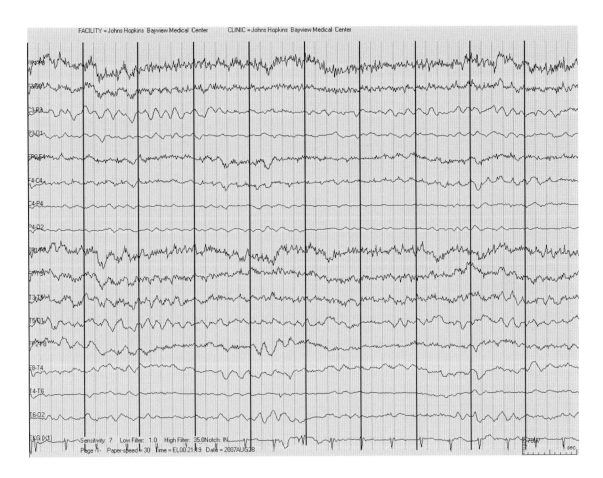

and autoimmune conditions, encephalitis, from adverse reactions to medications, and sudden withdrawal from benzodiazepines. It may be caused by decreased central dopaminergic activity from psychiatric, toxic, medical, or unknown origin.

PROGNOSIS: Chronic patients may survive with supportive care, but usually succumb to infection or organ failure. The underlying structural causes of VS are irreversible. Functional outcome given, these limitations can vary, and early in the course, patients may return to consciousness or emerge to a minimally conscious state. When VS has existed for a month, it is referred to as a *persistent* VS, and if present for 3 months after anoxia or 1 year after head trauma, it is regarded as permanent (PVS). These conditions are among the most distressing disorders seen in neurology, and the patient's family, physicians, and nurses may benefit from sensitive and extensive discussions. They may seek input from an ethics committee.

TREATMENT: Supportive care is usually initially provided in an ICU. With enduring states, when the patients may not require ventilation support, they can be supported in intermediate care units or high-level chronic care units.

In this patient in posttraumatic PVS, the EEG shows voltage suppression over the right hemisphere and diffuse monomorphic 4- to 6-Hz theta activity bilaterally.

REFERENCES:

1. Cartlidge N. States related to or confused with coma. *J Neurol Neurosurg Psychiatry* 2001;71(Supplement 1):i18–i19.
2. Laureys S, Owen AM, Schiff ND. Brain function in coma, vegetative state, and related disorders. *Lancet Neurol* 2004;3:557–546.
3. Young GB. Major syndromes of impaired consciousness. In: Young GB, Ropper AH, Bolton CF (eds.), *Coma and Impaired Consciousness: A Clinical Perspective.* New York: McGraw-Hill 1998:39–78.
4. Kaplan PW. Electrophysiological prognostication and brain injury from cardiac arrest. *Semin Neurol* 2006;26:403–412.

5. Teasdale G, Jennett B. Assessment of coma and impaired consciousness: A practical scale. *Lancet* 1974;2:81–84.

6. Booth CM, Boone RH, Tomlinson G, Detsky AS. Is this patient dead, vegetative, or severely neurologically impaired. *JAMA* 2004;291(7):870–879.

7. Fins JJ, Master MG, Gerber LM, Giacino JT. The minimally conscious state. *Arch Neruol* 2007;64(10):1400–1405.

8. Kampf A, Schmutzhard E, Franz G, Pfausler B, Haring H-P, Ulmer H, Felber S, Golaszewski S, Aichner F. Prediction of recovery from post-traumatic vegetative state with cerebral magnetic-resonance imaging. *Lancet* 1998;351:1763–1767.

9. Multi-Society Task Force on PVS. Medical aspects of the persistent vegetative state (first of two parts). *N Engl J Med* 1994;330:1499–1508.

10. Hansotia PL. Persistent vegetative state. *Arch Neurol* 1985;42:1048–1052.

11. Guérit JM, De Tourtchaninoff M, Soveges L, Mahieu P. The prognostic value of three-modality evoked potentials in evoked potentials (TMEPs) in anoxic and traumatic coma. *Neurophysiol Clin* 1993;23:209–226.

12. Scollo-Lavizzari G, Bassetti C. Prognostic value of EEG in post-anoxic coma after cardiac arrest. *Eur Neurol* 1987;26:161–170.

32. Minimally conscious state—after large, multifocal strokes [1–10]

NICU, CICU, MICU, SICU

CLINICAL CORRELATES: There is no purposeful limb or trunk reaction in response to outside command, and neither speech nor language. The eyes may be open, closed, or may open variably to sound, stimuli, or open spontaneously. Movement below the neck may be reflexive.

ETIOLOGY: It is most commonly seen after CRA, but can occur with strokes or head trauma. Coma is usually seen first. Minimally conscious state (MCS) can be seen with diffuse intracerebral edema associated with widespread ischemia from vascular compromise, and more rarely after drowning, carbon monoxide poisoning, hypotension, and/or anoxia during anesthesia. Also, it may occur after severe, diffuse encephalitis, and strokes producing bilateral frontal ischemia.

CLINICAL EVALUATION: Examine the brainstem reflexes and look for reactivity to stimuli. The clinical assessment is largely directed at determining if there is meaningful *yes/no* response to external stimuli. This indicates consciousness. Often, more prolonged observation is needed as families often report "meaningful" responses not seen by nurses and physicians. Assess the patient's score on the Glasgow coma scale (Table 29.1).

ANCILLARY TESTING: These states often trigger consults and requests for further investigations of "consciousness," "locked-in syndrome (LIS)," psychogenic unresponsiveness, or prognosis. Consider, in addition to, electrolytes and a toxin screen, somatosensory evoked potentials. A head CT or MRI may help to uncover the cause.

EEG: This patient had extensive postinfarction encephalomalacia in the right frontal, parietal, basal ganglia, and left frontal lobes.

Clinical Electrophysiology. By © Peter W. Kaplan and Thien Nguyen. Published 2011 Blackwell Publishing Ltd.

DIFFERENTIAL DIAGNOSIS

Coma—A clinical state of eyes-closed unresponsiveness from which the patient cannot be aroused (distinction from sleep) without purposeful response to external stimuli. If the cause is unknown, obtain a CT/MRI. If uninformative, look for toxic or metabolic causes.

Locked-in syndrome—De-efferented state: awake, conscious but minimal evidence of reaction (vertical/horizontal eye movements to questions). Imaging will usually show a stroke in or evidence of trauma to the midbrain/pontine area. Rarely, it occurs as an end-stage of severe, widespread peripheral paralysis (e.g., ALS, MG, and botulism). It occurs rarely in the ICU and OR in paralyzed patients (vecuronium, pancuronium) who are inadequately sedated or anesthetized.

Catatonia—A state of psychic and motor unresponsiveness. It is characterized by mutism, akinesia, and negativism and may be seen with schizophrenia, posttraumatic stress disorder, bipolar disease, depression, drug abuse, and overdose. It can occur with strokes, metabolic and autoimmune conditions, encephalitis, after severe adverse reactions to medications and sudden withdrawal from benzodiazepines. It may be caused by decreased central dopaminergic activity from psychiatric, toxic, medical, or unknown origin.

PROGNOSIS: Chronic patients may survive with supportive care, but usually succumb to infection or organ failure. The underlying structural causes of MCS are irreversible. Given these limitations, functional outcome can vary. Patients may return to vegetative state. The patient's family, physicians, and nurses may benefit from sensitive and extensive discussions. They may seek input from an ethics committee.

TREATMENT: Supportive care is usually initially provided in an ICU. With enduring states, when the patients may not require ventilation support, it can be provided

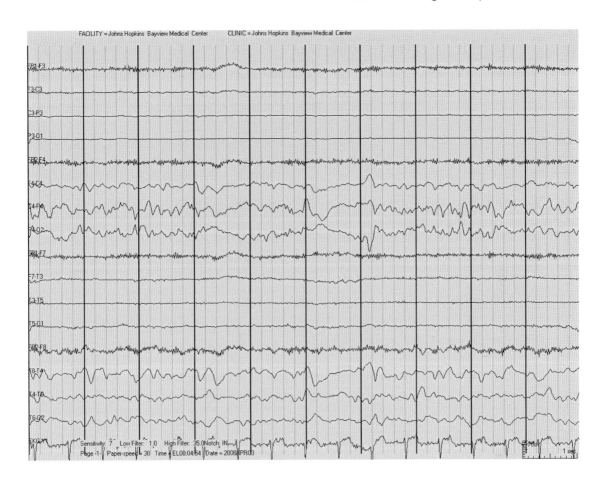

in intermediate care units or high-level chronic care units.

This EEG shows marked suppression over the left hemisphere and medium- to high-voltage mixed activity with slowing over the right hemisphere. As noted above, EEGs in patients with MCS can show a variety of patterns.

REFERENCES:

1. Kaplan PW. Electrophysiological prognostication and brain injury from cardiac arrest. *Semin Neurol* 2006;26:403–412.
2. Teasdale G, Jennett B. Assessment of coma and impaired consciousness: A practical scale. *Lancet* 1974;2:81–84.
3. Booth CM, Boone RH, Tomlinson G, Detsky AS. Is this patient dead, vegetative, or severely neurologically impaired. *JAMA* 2004;291(7):870–879.
4. Fins JJ, Master MG, Gerber LM, Giacino JT. The minimally conscious state. *Arch Neurol* 2007;64(10):1400–1405.
5. Kampf A, Schmutzhard E, Franz G, Pfausler B, Haring H-P, Ulmer H, Felber S, Golaszewski S, Aichner F. Prediction of recovery from post-traumatic vegetative state with cerebral magnetic-resonance imaging. *Lancet* 1998;351:1763–1767.
6. Guérit JM, De Tourtchaninoff M, Soveges L, Mahieu P. The prognostic value of three-modality evoked potentials in evoked potentials (TMEPs) in anoxic and traumatic coma. *Neurophysiol Clin* 1993;23:209–226.
7. Scollo-Lavizzari G, Bassetti C. Prognostic value of EEG in post-anoxic coma after cardiac arrest. *Eur Neurol* 1987;26:161–170.
8. Cartlidge N. States related to or confused with coma. *J Neurol Neurosurg Psychiatry* 2001;71(Supplement 1):i18–i19.
9. Laureys S, Owen AM, Schiff ND. Brain function in coma, vegetative state, and related disorders. *Lancet Neurol* 2004;3:557–546.
10. Young GB. Major syndromes of impaired consciousness. In: Young GB, Ropper AH, Bolton CF (eds.), *Coma and Impaired Consciousness: A Clinical Perspective*. New York: McGraw-Hill 1998:39–78.

33. Catatonia—psychogenic unresponsiveness/conversion disorder [1–5]

ER, Psychiatry

CLINICAL CORRELATES: Often the patients' eyes are closed and resist opening. Limb tone may be normal or increased without spasticity. There are few if any spontaneous limb movements, particularly when the patient is under direct observation. Reflexes are normal and there are no Babinski reflexes. Patients may not react to noxious stimuli. Brainstem reflexes are intact.

ETIOLOGY: These include psychogenic unresponsiveness with a conversion reaction. It is occasionally seen with malingerers or patients with Munchhausen syndrome. Organic causes include encephalitis, schizophrenia, and other psychiatric problems. Similar clinical states are seen with serotonin and neuroleptic malignant syndrome, and in nonconvulsive status epilepticus (NCSE).

CLINICAL EVALUATION: Look for eye opening and an inadvertent conjugate shift in gaze around the room. There may be stereotyped movements, rigidity, or loss of motor function. With catalepsy (waxy flexibility), patients can hold rigid and unusual poses for hours ("arm stays suspended in the air after the examiner lifts it up"). The patient may resist movement (*gegenhalten*). There may be nonsense speech or repeat statements. Avoid painful stimuli beyond routine noxious input such as from saline drops to elicit corneal responses, cotton swab for intranasal stimulation to look for facial grimacing, and plantar responses. Deep nail-bed pressure is unwarranted. In unclear cases, caloric stimulation has been used.

ANCILLARY TESTING: Usually the diagnosis is suspected. For unclear cases, assess for the other clinical states, and thence the respective underlying etiologies. In atypical cases of drug toxicity or encephalitis, tests for these should be considered. Imaging is rarely informative. Sodium amytal "interview" has been used in the past. For the differential diagnosis of serotonin or neuroleptic malignant syndromes, consider obtaining a toxin screen, CPK, and liver enzymes. Suggest a psychiatry consultation.

DIFFERENTIAL DIAGNOSIS:

Some operational definitions of other states of prolonged unresponsiveness are as follows:

Coma—A clinical state of eyes-closed unresponsiveness from which the patient cannot be aroused (distinction from sleep) without purposeful response to external stimuli.

Vegetative state—Awake (eyes open) but unconscious.

Locked-in syndrome—De-efferented state: awake, conscious, but minimal evidence of reaction to external input (vertical or horizontal eye movements to questions).

Clinical—Consider neuroleptic malignant syndrome, serotonin syndrome, lithium, baclofen toxicity, NCSE. Also, think of locked-in-syndrome, persistent vegetative state, or a minimally conscious state.

EEG—The EEG in psychogenic cases shows a reactive waking alpha pattern. In NCSE, there is seizure activity on the EEG. Periodic lateralized epileptiform discharges and other periodic discharges may be seen with encephalitis, multifocal brain disease, recent seizures, and confusional states after a stroke or structural brain lesion with seizures. Patients with encephalitis may show diffuse slow EEG activity. Drug toxicities and the neuroleptic malignant syndrome may have triphasic waves on EEG. Some cases of conversion reaction or psychogenic unresponsiveness respond to benzodiazepines, amobarbital, or zolpidem.

Clinical Electrophysiology. By © Peter W. Kaplan and Thien Nguyen. Published 2011 Blackwell Publishing Ltd.

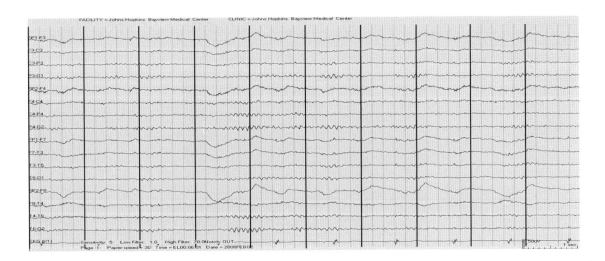

DISCUSSION: Patients with psychogenic unresponsiveness often trigger neurology consults. As noted above, although there are varying levels of cooperation and response to external cues, the patient may exhibit waxy rigidity, be strikingly impervious to stimuli, but occasionally show rapid directed conjugate eye movements.

This EEG shows normal waking, posterior, alpha activity that is reactive to eye opening and closure.

REFERENCES:

1. Valenstein M, Maltbie A, Kaplan PW. Catatonia in the ED. *Ann Emerg Med* 1985;14:359–361.

2. Bush G, Fink M, Petrides G, Dowling F, Francis A. Catatonia II. Treatment with lorazepam and electroconvulsive therapy. *Acta Psychiatr Scand* 1996;93:137–43.

3. Swartz CM, Bottum KM, Salazar LS. Suppression of catatonia-like signs by lorazepam in nonconvulsive status epilepticus without seizure termination. *Am J Geriatr Psychiatry* 2002;10:348–350.

4. Ono Y, Manabe Y, Hamakawa Y, Omori N, Abe K. Steroid-responsive encephalitis lethargic with malignant catatonia. *Intern Med* 2007;46:307–310.

5. Suzuki K, Miura N, Awata S, Ebina Y, Takano T, Honda T, Shindo T, Matsuoka H. Epileptic seizures superimposed on catatonic stupor. *Epilepsia* 2006;47:793–798.

34. Somatosensory evoked potential prognosis in anoxic coma [1–8]

CICU, MICU, Burns ICU, SICU, Ward

CLINICAL CORRELATES: When somatosensory evoked potentials (SSEPs) are used for prognosis, the patient should be in coma, and have no purposeful movement or posturing. There may be preservation or absence of brainstem reflexes.

ETIOLOGY: For prognostication, SSEPs are most reliable after CRA/anoxia and then after head trauma.

CLINICAL EVALUATION: Examine brainstem reflexes and assess Glasgow coma scale. Obtain cause of coma.

ANCILLARY TESTING: EEG, CT, or MRI; protein S-100B (S-100B); neuron-specific enolase. Consider toxicology screen, although benzodiazepines rarely suppress cortical responses completely.

DIFFERENTIAL DIAGNOSIS: Clinical context is paramount. The absolute prognostic value lies only with CRA or anoxia. The value in head trauma is less absolute—see below. Ensure that the patient is in coma and ascertain the cause before providing clinical correlation and prognosis. Severe nonstructural causes of coma may impair cortical SSEP responses. Also, mechanical interruption of ascending SSEP volley may occur at the cervical level in an awake patient, as may severe peripheral neuropathies (e.g., diabetic).

PROGNOSIS: SSEPs are often used after EEG and in concert with the clinical examination to provide clinical information on the degree of anatomic pathway impairment, and to provide prognosis.

a. In post-CRA/anoxic coma, meta-analysis has confirmed the 100% predictive value of a negative out-come (persistent vegetative state or death) if N20s are absent. See above caveats.

b. For head trauma, prognosis is unclear. Some patients may recover [2], but absent N20 still indicates a poor outcome—100% if bilaterally absent. Conversely, a bilaterally normal SSEP and brainstem auditory evoked potentials (BAEP) indicated a Glasgow outcome score of 4 or 5 (good outcome) with a positive predictive value of 98% in 100 patients [3]. Cortical N20 prolongation progressively occurs with brainstem herniation from raised Intracranial pressure (ICP) [5]; others disagree.

c. In central nervous system-depressant drug poisoning (overdose with amitriptyline, meprobamate, barbiturates, and nitrazepam), N20 can be delayed and dispersed, but not abolished, and distinguishes toxic from "therapeutic" coma [4].

d. With anesthesia (propofol, isoflurane, and nitrous oxide), N20 amplitudes may be reduced, but are not abolished [6].

e. In nonanoxic, nonstructural coma, prognosis is highly variable, but better than trauma or anoxia; data are few. Hepatic coma, with cerebral edema and a raised ICP, abolished the cortical N20, with a fatal outcome [7].

f. In poor-grade subarachnoid hemorrhage (SAH) patients after aneurismal surgery, bilateral N20 absence was fatal [8].

This SSEP study shows a peripheral response from the stimulus, a response at Erb's point (as the afferent volley goes past the recording electrode—N9), a near-field potential N13 as the impulse enters and turns cephalad at the cervical dorsal route entry zone, and subcortical (far-field) P13/N18 potentials probably arising from thalamic or thalamocortical structures. There is *no* cortical N-20 potential after stimulation of each side. This indicates absence of cortical somatosensory activity.

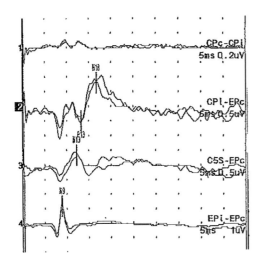
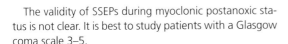
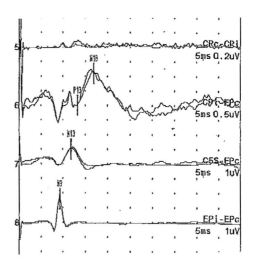

The validity of SSEPs during myoclonic postanoxic status is not clear. It is best to study patients with a Glasgow coma scale 3–5.

REFERENCES:

1. Wijdicks EFM, Hijdra A, Young GB, Bassetti CL, Wiebe S. Practice parameter: prediction of outcome in comatose survivors after cardiopulmonary resuscitation (an evidence-based review): Report of the quality standards subcommittee of the American Academy of Neurology. *Neurology* 2006;67:203–210.

2. Sleigh JW, Havill JH, Frith R, Kersel D, Marsh N, Ulyatt D. SSEPs in severe traumatic brain injury: A blinded study. *J Neurosurg* 1999;91:577–580.

3. Morgalla MH, Bauer J, Ritz R, Tatagiba M. Coma. The prognostic value of evoked potentials in patients with traumatic brain injury (in German). *Anaesthesist* 2006;55:760–768.

4. Rumpl E, Prugger M, Battista HJ, Badry F, Gerstenbrand F, Dienstl F. Short latency SSEPs and BAEPs in coma due to CNS depressant drug poisoning. *Electroencephalogr Clin Neurophysiol* 1988;70:482–489.

5. Reisecker F, Witzmann A, Loffler W, Lebhuber F, Deisenhammer E, Valencak E. SSEPs in comatose patients: Comparison with clinical findings, EEG and prognosis. *EEG EMG Z Elektroenzephalogr Elektromyogr Verwandte Geb* 1985;16(2):87–92.

6. Clapcich A, Emerson RG, Roye D, Xie H, Gallo EJ, Dowling KC, Ramnath B, Heyer EJ. The effects of propofol, small-dose isoflurane and nitrous oxide on ortical somatosensory evoked potential and bispectral index monitoring in adolescents undergoing spinal fusion. *Anesth Analg* 2004;99:1334–1340.

7. Yang SS, Chu NS, Wu CH. Disappearance of N20 and P25 components of SSEP and ominous sign in severe acute hepatitis. *J Formos Med Assoc* 1993;92:46–49.

8. Ritz R, Schwerdtfeger K, Strowitzki M, Donauer E, Koenig J, Steudel WI. Prognostic value of SSEP in early aneurysm surgery after SAH in poor grade patients. *Neurol Res* 2002;24:756–764.

35. Somatosensory evoked potential prognosis in head trauma

NICU, MICU, SICU

CLINICAL CORRELATES: For coma prognosis the patient should be in coma, eyes-closed, and have no purposeful movement. There may be posturing and preservation or absence of brainstem reflexes.

ETIOLOGY: Head trauma.

CLINICAL EVALUATION: Examine brainstem reflexes and assess Glasgow coma scale. Obtain cause of coma.

ANCILLARY TESTING: EEG, CT, or MRI for review of the extent of central nervous system trauma, herniation, and edema. Consider tox screen.

CLINICAL CONSIDERATIONS: After closed head injury (CHI), there are various combinations of somatosensory evoked potential (SSEP) abnormality, sustained from direct and countercoup cerebral and brain stem injury, brain edema, intracerebral, subdural and subarachnoid hemorrhage, diffuse axonal injury (DAI), effects of anesthesia, spinal cord trauma and loss of peripheral SSEP input from peripheral nerve, brachial plexus, and afferent radicular avulsion. Close clinical correlation is needed to avoid over-interpretation of SSEP deficits.

DIFFERENTIAL DIAGNOSIS: Clinical context is paramount. Ensure that technical and peripheral factors do not account for absent responses, for example, avulsion of nerve routes, cervical compromise (tetraplegia). Determine if the accident was unwitnessed, whether hypoxia and hypotension might have occurred (see coma with anoxia). Anesthetics and sedatives prolong N20 latencies but do not abolish them.

PROGNOSIS [1–5]**:** Cortical responses may be obtained down to a core body temperature of 28°C. A reliable absolute prognostic value of SSEPs with head trauma (without anoxia or hypotension) is seen only with sustained bilateral absence of N20 potentials (poor outcome), or conversely a preserved N20 with little prolongation. Sustained bilaterally absent N20 has been reported to be 100% poor outcome [3]. Good Glasgow outcome score is seen with bilaterally normal SSEPs and BAEPs (positive predictive value 98% in 100 patients) [1]. Reversible, bilateral absence of cortical potentials can occur from a circumscribed contusion [2], but is rare. Initial SSEPs correlate with long-term outcome in CHI with DAI—bilateral absent N20s predicted death in 100% [4]. Blinded and unblinded studies support this prognostic value [3,4]. N20 prolongation progressively occurs with brainstem herniation from raised ICP [5]; others report that ICP does not cause SSEP deterioration, but that it is due to deterioration of brain function.

This SSEP study shows a peripheral response from the stimulus at the wrist, a response at Erb's point (as the afferent volley goes past the recording electrode—N9), a near-field potential N13 as the impulse enters and turns cephalad at the cervical dorsal route entry zone, and subcortical (far-field) P14/N18 potentials probably arising from thalamic or thalamocortical structures.

Clinical Electrophysiology. By © Peter W. Kaplan and Thien Nguyen.
Published 2011 Blackwell Publishing Ltd.

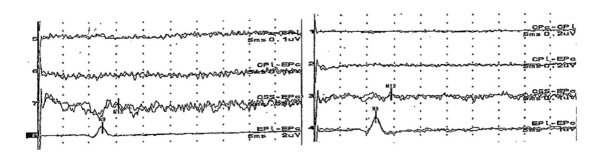

REFERENCES:

1. Morgalla MH, Bauer J, Ritz R, Tatagiba M. Coma. The prognostic value of evoked potentials in patients with traumatic brain injury (in German). *Anaesthesist* 2006;55:760–768.
2. Pohlmann-Eden B, Dingenthal K, Bender HJ, Koelfen W. How reliable is the predictive value of SEP patterns in severe brain damage with special regard to the bilateral loss of cortical responses? *Int Care Med* 1997;23:301–318.
3. Sleigh JW, Havill JH, Frith R. Kersel D, Marsh N, Ulyatt D. SSEPs in severe traumatic brain injury: A blinded study. *J Neurosurg* 1999;91:577–580.
4. Claassen J, Hansen H-C. Early recovery after closed traumatic head injury: SSEPs and clinical findings. *Crit Care Med* 2001;29:494–502.
5. Konasiewicz SJ, Moulton RJ, Shedden PM. SSEPs and ICP in severe head injury. *Can J Neurol Sci* 1994;21:219–226.

Section C: Evoked potentials in consultative neurology

Evoked potentials involve laboratory or bedside testing of central nervous system function by stimulating end-organs (for vision, hearing, or sensation) and collecting summated averages of the brain's responses.

Visual evoked potentials

Visual evoked potentials (VEPs) are the easiest, take less than 20 minutes in the cooperative patient, and can be used to detect demyelination in vision from one or the other eye. In hysterical blindness, VEPs can establish (even in an uncooperative patient with closed eyelids) that light can travel from each eye to the visual cortex, and this test too can take less than an hour. Longer latency cognitive potentials are more difficult to set up and are little used clinically at present.

Brainstem auditory evoked potentials

Brainstem auditory evoked potentials (BAEPs) delivers "clicks" or tones via tubal ear inserts or headphones to the eardrum. These studies can also assess brainstem demyelination and have been used to assess potential survivability from irreversibility or partially reversible damage to the brainstem from anoxia, cardiac arrest, or trauma. In this function, they are less used than are somatosensory evoked potentials (SSEPs). If all responses beyond wave I are absent in a comatose patient after cardiac arrest without known deafness or peripheral hearing loss, they are a reliable prognostic indicator of death or persistent vegetative state (PVS).

BAEPs using longer latency responses at about 70 or 100 ms after the auditory stimulus, "oddball" stimuli, or mismatched negativity are being increasingly studied.

In these paradigms the time window for summated and averaged acquisition is lengthened to encompass these delayed responses. Because these potentials probably represent higher orders of cognitive processing (and awareness), they are being explored as surrogates of consciousness or awareness. Investigators have found them to be useful in differentiating awake patients after underwater anoxia who may either evolve to consciousness or conversely remain in a PVS.

Somatosensory evoked potentials

SSEPs, typically responses obtained from median nerve stimulation (in the arm), can be used to delineate where there is a peripheral interruption of input at the brachial plexus in plexus avulsion (trauma), for investigating pyramidal pathway impairment in the neck and brainstem, and to test for possible demyelination along the ascending somatosensory pathway. Perhaps most frequently in the inpatient hospital setting, SSEPs are used to evaluate prognosis after anoxic coma.

In coma, SSEPs play a special role in firmly establishing a poor or negative outcome. After CRA, the absence of cortical responses accurately predicts a nonreturn to consciousness with 100% accuracy. Unconscious patients may deteriorate and die, or enter an unconscious vegetative state. Outcome after head trauma can also be assessed accurately with SSEPs. Conversely, and not surprisingly, reversible causes of coma are not prognosticated well by this test—cortical responses in SSEPs persist in comatose, anesthetized patients and many patients with toxic or metabolic coma.

The handbook will examine particular patient "scenarios" and problems that would prompt neurological consultation, and meld in the electrophysiological findings into a diagnosis or prognosis where most applicable.

36. Somatosensory evoked potentials in midbrain lesion—absent cortical responses

CLINICAL CASE: A 44-year-old woman with hypertension, severe headache, and seizures became unresponsive to stimuli. Examination revealed a comatose patient, with closed eyes, and pupils fixed at 5 mm. There were no doll's eyes responses, corneal reflexes, response to nasal stimulation or gag, and no spontaneous respiration. Imaging revealed an intracerebral hemorrhage in the pons and midbrain.

COMMENT: With the absence of most brainstem reflexes, the presence of an irreversible cause of coma, and SSEPs showing no conduction beyond the midbrain, the intensive care physicians met with the family. Together they elected to withdraw care.

Clinical Electrophysiology. By © Peter W. Kaplan and Thien Nguyen.
Published 2011 Blackwell Publishing Ltd.

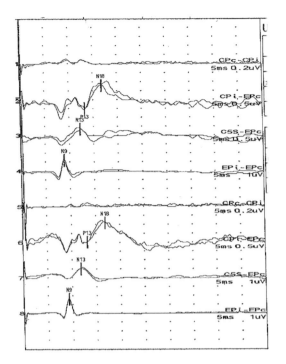

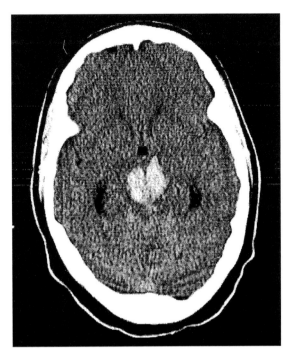

This median nerve SSEP shows evidence of bilateral ascending somatosensory signal through the brachial plexus Erb's point (N9), progressing through the cervical dorsal root entry zone (N13), and producing evidence of far-field projections from subcortical, medial lemniscal somatosensory regions (P13/N18). There was no evidence of further signal reaching the somatosensory cortex (absent N20). This corresponded to the CT head scan, which showed an intracranial hemorrhage in the midbrain and pons.

37. Somatosensory evoked potentials in diffuse cortical anoxic injury—absent cortical and subcortical responses [1]

CLINICAL CASE: A 26-year-old woman was found in cardiac arrest after a drug overdose. She was pulseless, apneic, and had dilated pupils. In the ICU, examination revealed no spontaneous or evoked movements and she had no brainstem reflexes.

COMMENT: With the absence of brainstem reflexes, with a history of a documented anoxic/ischemic cause of coma, and with evidence from median nerve somatosensory evoked potentials (SSEPs) showing no conduction to cortical structures above the midbrain (absent N20 responses), there was no possibility of return to consciousness. The intensive care physicians met with the family who elected to withdraw care.

Clinical Electrophysiology. By © Peter W. Kaplan and Thien Nguyen.
Published 2011 Blackwell Publishing Ltd.

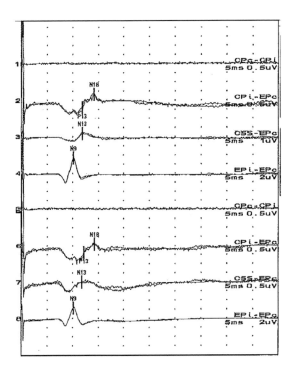

This median nerve SSEP shows evidence of bilateral ascending somatosensory signal through the brachial plexus (N9), progressing through the cervical dorsal root entry zone (N13), and evidence of far-field projections from subcortical, medial lemniscus somatosensory regions (P14/N18), but no evidence of the stimulus reaching the somatosensory cortex (absent N20).

The EEG showed spindle activity over the frontal regions bilaterally.

REFERENCE:

1. Zandbergen EGJ, Hijdra A, Koelman JHTM, Hart AAM, Vos PE, Verbeek MM, de Haan RJ. Prediction of poor outcome within the first three days of post anoxic coma. *Neurology* 2006;66:62–68.

38. Somatosensory evoked potentials in prolonged cardiac arrest—absence of all waves above the brachial plexus [1, 2]

CLINICAL CASE: A 52-year-old man was found in asystolic cardiac arrest after a drug overdose. In the cardiac intensive care unit (CICU), examination revealed no spontaneous or evoked movements, and no brainstem reflexes.

COMMENT: This patient had no evidence of cortical or brainstem function by clinical examination. The absence of cortical responses on median nerve somatosensory evoked potentials (SSEPs) helped the family come to a decision with the CICU physicians on the withdrawal of care. Absent SSEP cortical responses appear to play a key role in the decision-making process for withdrawal of care.

Clinical Electrophysiology. By © Peter W. Kaplan and Thien Nguyen.
Published 2011 Blackwell Publishing Ltd.

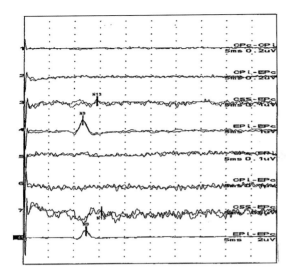

This median nerve SSEP shows evidence of bilateral ascending somatosensory signals only through the brachial plexus at Erb's point (N9) and the cervical dorsal root entry zone (N13) on the left. In contrast to the prior study, there is no evidence of conduction through subcortical or cortical regions (neither P14/N18, nor N20 responses). On the right, there is no conduction above the brachial plexus under Erb's point.

REFERENCES

1. Zandbergen EGJ, Hijdra A, Koelman JHTM, Hart AAM, Vos PE, Verbeek MM, de Haan RJ. Prediction of poor outcome within the first three days of post-anoxic coma. *Neurology* 2006;66:62–68.
2. Geocadin RG, Buitrago M, Torbey MT, Chandra-Strobos N, Williams A, Kaplan PW. Neurological prognostication and withdrawal of life sustaining therapies in patients resuscitated from cardiac arrest. *Neurology* 2006;67:105–108.

39. Somatosensory evoked potentials after prolonged cardiac arrest—absence of all responses except cervical N9 [1, 2]

CLINICAL CASE: A 36-year-old man with cardiac disease had a pulseless cardiac arrest. In the ICU, he had no brainstem reflexes, no response to noxious stimuli, and no spontaneous movements. Head CT showed marked diffuse cerebral edema with effacement of all cerebral and cerebellar sulci, superior spinal canal, fourth ventricle, and tectal and suprasellar cisterns. The EEG showed a Grade V pattern postanoxic coma grade, with little if any low-voltage cortical activity, at 2–4 μV.

COMMENT: With the absence of brainstem reflexes, a documented anoxic/ischemic cause of coma, and somatosensory evoked potentials (SSEPs) showing no responses above the brachial plexus, the probability for return to consciousness was zero. In this study, all conduction above the cervical dorsal root entry zone was abolished. The intensive care physicians met with the family, who elected to withdraw care.

Clinical Electrophysiology. By © Peter W. Kaplan and Thien Nguyen.
Published 2011 Blackwell Publishing Ltd.

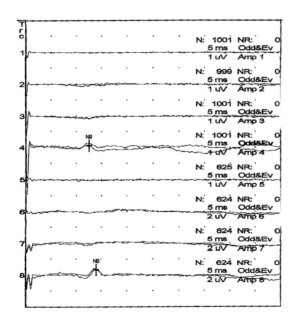

This median nerve SSEP shows evidence bilaterally of ascending somatosensory signal through the brachial plexus (N9) only. There is no evidence of signal through structures cephalad to the brachial plexus. Hence, there was no response from the cervical dorsal root entry zone, subcortical and cortical somatosensory pathways.

REFERENCES:

1. Zandbergen EGJ, Hijdra A, Koelman JHTM, Hart AAM, Vos PE, Verbeek MM, de Haan RJ. Prediction of poor outcome within the first three days of post anoxic coma. *Neurology* 2006;66:62–68.
2. Scollo-Lavizzari G, Bassetti C. Prognostic value of EEG in post-anoxic coma after cardiac arrest. *Eur Neurol* 1987;26:161–170.

40. Somatosensory evoked potentials—median and tibial after traumatic spinal cord injury

CLINICAL CASE: A 22-year-old woman sustained a gunshot wound to the neck. Examination revealed a flaccid tetraplegia, retained facial and neck muscle movements, and the absence of sensation below the neck. The head CT was normal. Neck CT revealed a hematoma and bone fragments in the vertebral canal at C5. A neck CT angiogram showed patent vertebral and carotid arteries without evidence of arterial dissection.

COMMENT: Together, these studies revealed the total somatosensory interruption in the neck, consistent with the flaccid tetraplegia. Surgery was not attempted.

Clinical Electrophysiology. By © Peter W. Kaplan and Thien Nguyen.
Published 2011 Blackwell Publishing Ltd.

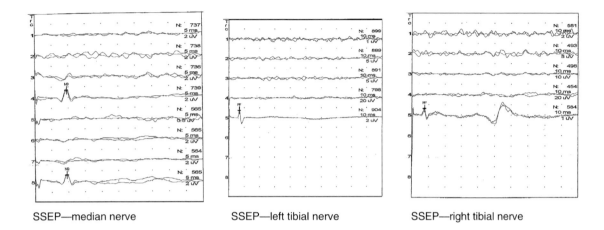

SSEP—median nerve   SSEP—left tibial nerve   SSEP—right tibial nerve

This set of median nerve somatosensory evoked potentials (SSEPs) shows no evidence (bilaterally) of ascending somatosensory signal beyond the brachial plexus (N9). The tibial nerve SSEP also revealed no evidence of re- sponses cephalad to the popliteal fossa (PF); lumbar (LP) potentials could not be obtained. Together, the studies reflect the total transection of cuneate and gracile as- cending somatosensory pathways in the neck.

41. Visual evoked potentials in worsening vision

CLINICAL CASE: A patient with a prior history sugges-tive of multiple sclerosis and several episodes of relapsing and remitting neurological symptoms noted the suba-cute onset of blurring of vision in her right eye. Examina-tion revealed right optic disc pallor and diminished visual acuity.

COMMENT: Visual evoked potentials (VEPs) have found their principal use in the documentation of demyelina-tion in the anterior optic pathway in multiple sclerosis (MS) [1]. Papilledema typically does not produce changes in latency or amplitude unless there is actual or pend-ing visual loss. Compression of the anterior visual path-ways and intrinsic optic nerve tumors may distort the VEP waveform morphology, but usually produces less latency delay than with demyelination [2, 3]. Clearly, the best testing modality for such lesions is MRI. Several other dis-eases may have inconsistent findings, including albinism (decreased amplitude, but without latency change), al-coholism and Wernicke–Korsakoff syndrome, and pro-longation in chronic demyelinating polyradiculopathy [4]. Some delay in patients with diabetes may be resemble the changes seen in MS. Head injury and raised intracranial pressure may also affect VEPs [4], but VEPs have not been used much for these problems. VEPs can be used to moni-tor leukodystrophies. With adrenoleukodystrophy [5] and vitamin E deficiency in cystic fibrosis [6], VEPs have been used to monitor worsening, or conversely, the improve-ment with therapy. A cortical response after stimulation with light-emitting diode goggles may be helpful in the diagnosis (or not) of hysterical blindness.

This VEP, performed with small and then large check sizes, demonstrates delayed latencies of the P100 to 120–122 ms on the right, compared with 99–100 ms on the left, with a laboratory norm of 108 ms ±3 SDs. The right side is clearly delayed, reflecting demyelination of the right anterior optic pathway (consistent with right optic neuritis and a recurrence of MS).

REFERENCES:

1. Brooks EB, Chiappa KH. A comparison of clinical neuro-ophthalmological findings, and pattern-shift visual evoked potentials in multiple sclerosis In: Courjon J, Maugiere F, Revol M (eds.), *Clinical Applications of Evoked Potentials in Neurol-ogy*. New York: Raven Press 1982.
2. Kupersmith MJ, Siegel IM, Carr RE, Ransohoff J, Flamm E, Shakin E. Visual evoked potentials in chiasmal gliomas in four adults. *Arch Neurol* 1981;38:362–365.
3. Haliday AM, McDonald WI, Mushin J. Visual evoked re-sponses in the diagnosis of multiple sclerosis. *Br Med J* 1973;4:661–664.
4. Chiappa KH (ed.), *Evoked Potentials in Clinical Medicine*, 2nd edn. New York: Raven Press 1990;645.
5. Kaplan PW, Tusa RJ, Shankroff J, Heller J, Moser HW. Visual evoked potentials in adrenoleukodystrophy: A trial with glyc-erol trioleate and lorenzo oil. *Ann Neurol* 1993;34:169–174.
6. Kaplan PW, Rawal K, Erwin CW, D'Souza BJ, Spock A. Vi-sual and somatosensory evoked potentials in vitamin E de-ficiency with cystic fibrosis. *Electroencephalogr Clin Neuro-physiol* 1988;71:266–272.

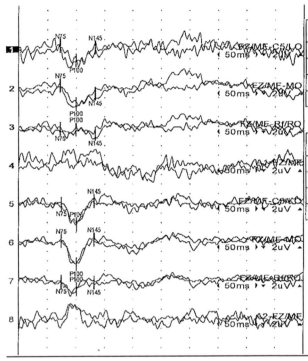

Left VEP measurements

Text	Lat N75 ms	Lat P100 ms	Lat N145 ms	PP Amp 75-100 uV
	1.1 N75	1.1 P100	1.1 N145	1.1 N75 P100
LO	70.5	99.0	133	3.15
	12 N75	12 P100	12 N145	12 N75 P100
MO	70.5	99.0	133	3.92
	13 N75	13 P100	13 N145	13 N75 P100
RO	70.5	99.0	133	0.06
		1.4 N100		
MF				

Left VEP measurements

Text	Lat N75 ms	Lat P100 ms	Lat N145 ms	PP Amp 75-100 uV
	2.1 N75	2.1 P100	2.1 N145	2.1 N75 P100
RO	72.5	100	131	4.06
	22 N75	22 P100	22 N145	22 N75 P100
MO	72.5	100	131	4.96
	23 N75	23 P100	23 N145	23 N75 P100
LO	72.5	100	131	1.51
		2.4 N100		
MF				

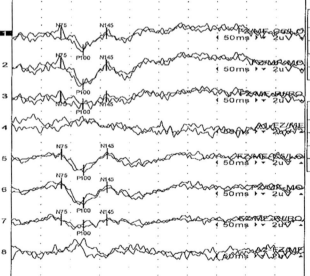

Right VEP measurements

Text	Lat N75 ms	Lat P100 ms	Lat N145 ms	PP Amp 75-100 uV
	1.1 N75	1.1 P100	1.1 N145	1.1 N75 P100
LO	81.5	120	160	4.56
	12 N75	12 P100	12 N145	12 N75 P100
MO	81.5	120	160	5.73
	13 N75	13 P100	13 N145	13 N75 P100
RO	81.5	120	160	2.05
		1.4 N100		
MF				

Right VEP measurements

Text	Lat N75 ms	Lat P100 ms	Lat N145 ms	PP Amp 75-100 uV
	2.1 N75	2.1 P100	2.1 N145	2.1 N75 P100
RO	83.5	122	162	4.37
	22 N75	22 P100	22 N145	22 N75 P100
MO	83.5	122	162	5.09
	23 N75	23 P100	23 N145	23 N75 P100
LO	83.5	122	162	1.63
		2.4 N100		
MF				

42. Brainstem auditory evoked potentials—in worsening hearing

CLINICAL CASE: A patient with a history of multiple sclerosis and episodes of relapsing and remitting neurologic problems complained of sudden decrease in hearing on the left. Examination revealed decreased perception of noise in the left ear.

COMMENT: Brainstem auditory evoked potentials (BAEPs) have been used in evaluation of cerebellopontine angle tumors, acoustic neuromas, intrinsic brain stem lesions, and MS. For these indications, BAEPs have largely been superceded by brain MRI. In addition to other audiologic tests, BAEPs have been useful in evaluating the effects of ototoxic drugs.

In coma and brain death, BAEPs are used to supplement the clinical examination and other electrophysiological studies, such as somatosensory evoked potentials and the EEG. Regarding hearing, peripheral causes (cochlear and 8th nerve disorders) have little effect on BAEP latencies. In MS, BAEP abnormalities are often associated with normal hearing. In one series, 45% of MS patients with abnormal BAEPs had unilateral BAEP abnormalities [1], usually ipsilateral to the side of the lesion. With all the above caveats, BAERs can be used to document or investigate *changes* in waveforms, thus reflecting quantitative function changes in the brainstem peripheral and central auditory pathways. Wave I–III delay is most sensitive to acoustic neuromas, and if normal can obviate a brain MRI [2]. In MS patients with nonbrainstem disease manifestations, BAEPs when abnormal can help by signaling abnormalities in the brainstem, thus helping further define the disease and signal multiple anatomical disease sites. If the clinical history, imaging, or cerebrospinal fluid is inconclusive, BAEPs might indicate objective evidence of brainstem involvement.

Finally, BAEPs enable the monitoring of treatment effects or disease progression. With MS, most abnormalities involve wave V amplitude (87% of cases), the II–V interval (superior olivary nucleus and inferior colliculus). Occasionally, rarefraction clicks can distinguish affected cases [3]. BAEPs may follow the clinical progression/regression of central pontine myelinolysis [4], metachromatic and adrenoleukodystrophy, Pelizaeus–Merzbacher disease, and other hereditary degenerative central nervous system disorders [2], and may help (when normal) distinguish toxic/metabolic coma from brainstem causes.

In head injury and raised intracranial pressure, BAEPs have had variable success among different patient series in predicting outcome. In suspected severe brain dysfunction, BAEPs may be used to follow comatose patients in whom anesthetic agents or raised ICPs complicate the interpretation of the clinical comatose state [4].

In infants, BAEPs are used as a screening tool for hearing defects in infants at-risk, such as after bacterial meningitis, exposure to ototoxic drugs, kernicterus, and prematurity. Testing has been advocated on all ICU infants prior to discharge and in developmentally delayed infants and children who may be blind or deaf.

Clinical Electrophysiology. By © Peter W. Kaplan and Thien Nguyen.
Published 2011 Blackwell Publishing Ltd.

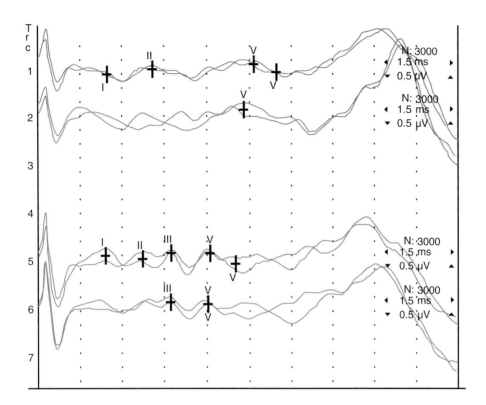

This BAEP shows normal peaks I–V ipsilateral to the right ear stimulation (bottom two tracings). On the left (upper two traces), the peaks are less well defined, peak III is not seen, and there is prolongation of the I–V interpeak interval. This indicates prolongation in the pons-midbrain region. These results support brainstem demyelination as the locus for hearing loss and hence a further exacerbation of MS.

REFERENCES:

1. Chiappa KH, Harrison JL, Brooks EB, Young RR. Brainstem auditory evoked responses in 200 patients with multiple sclerosis. *Ann Neurol* 1980;7:135–143.

2. Chiappa KH. *Evoked Potentials in Clinical Medicine*, 2nd edn. New York: Raven Press 1990.

3. Emerson RG, Brooks EB, Parker SW, Chiappa KH. Effects of click polarity on brainstem auditory evoked potentials in normal subjects and patients: Unexpected sensitivity of wave V. *Ann N Y Acad Sci* 1982;388:710–721.

4. Stockard JJ, Sharbrough FW. Unique contributions of short-latency somatosensory evoked potentials in patients with neurological lesions. *Prog Clin Neurophysiol* 1980;7:231–263.

PART 4
Peripheral nervous system disease

Section A: Weakness and/or respiratory failure in ICU and on the ward

Generalized somatic weakness and respiratory failure are common manifestations of neuromuscular disorders in the ICU and on the ward. Weakness has a wide differential diagnosis and may present a major challenge to the consulting clinician. The most common ICU-acquired neuromuscular disorder is critical illness neuromyopathy (Case 43), while prolonged neuromuscular junction blockade and rhabdomyolysis are fairly rare causes. Other neuromuscular disorders such as myasthenia gravis, motor neuron diseases, and inflammatory myopathies may cause weakness in ICU patients, but these and other similar disorders often occur outside the ICU and may eventually lead to ICU admission. In floor patients, weakness and respiratory failure usually involves neuropathies, radiculopathies and less frequently myopathy, myositis, vasculitis, and the effects of malignancy. ALS is not rare. Nonetheless, most floor consults are on patients with weakness after prolonged illness due to general debility, bed rest, and lack of mobility. A careful, detailed medical history and examination are essential to diagnosing neuromuscular disorders and the proper interpretation of ancillary tests such as electrodiagnostic studies. The goals are to determine whether the disease is acquired or inherited, to identify whether the process is focal (i.e., mononeuropathies or radiculopathies) or generalized (polyneuropathies or myopathies), and to localize the affected neurologic regions (i.e., brain/spinal cord, nerve root, plexus, nerve, neuromuscular junction, or muscle). A systematic approach to the neurological examination is crucial to discerning these details and is discussed below. Physical findings seen in various neurological disorders are summarized in Case 44.

Cranial nerve involvement can be helpful in narrowing the differential diagnoses. Cranial nerve dysfunction is common in neuromuscular transmission disorders (i.e., diplopia, ptosis, dysarthria, dysphagia, and bilateral facial weakness in myasthenia gravis) and motor neuron diseases (i.e., dysarthria, dysphagia, and tongue weakness in ALS). It is rare in neuropathies (with the exception of bilateral facial weakness in patients with Guillain-Barré syndrome) and myopathies (with the exception of bilateral facial weakness which occurs in myotonic dystrophy and ophthalmoplegia in oculopharyngeal dystrophies and mitochondrial disorders).

Bedside manual muscle testing should always be performed and quantitated. The pattern of muscle weakness may be helpful. Weakness is proximal in most myopathies and some motor neuron diseases, but it is distal in most polyneuropathies. Ptosis and extraocular weakness are seen in myasthenia gravis, oculopharyngeal dystrophy, and mitochondrial myopathies. Facial weakness is characteristic of facioscapulohumeral dystrophy, but may be seen in sarcoidosis or familial amyloidosis. Tongue weakness with atrophy and fasciculation occurs in motor neuron disease. Tongue weakness without fasciculations may occur in myasthenia gravis.

Muscle testing should try to determine whether weakness is accompanied by focal or generalized atrophy, or whether there is lack of muscle atrophy. Neuromuscular transmission disorders and demyelinating neuropathies usually do not cause muscle atrophy. Muscle fatigue during repetitive motion suggests neuromuscular transmission disorders, although it can also occur in other diseases.

Increased muscle tendon reflexes or hyperreflexia indicates upper motor neuron dysfunction, as seen in spinal cord lesions and motor neuron diseases. Hyporeflexia indicates neuropathy, but may also be seen in Lambert-Eaton myasthenic syndrome and lower motor neuron forms of motor neuron diseases. Distal areflexia is characteristic of axonal neuropathies, but generalized areflexia points to a demyelinating process. Hyporeflexia that improves during repetitive motion can be observed in Lambert-Eaton myasthenic syndrome. A focal reflex loss with sensory deficit suggests a lesion in a particular nerve, plexus, or root. Reflexes are generally normal in myopathies.

Sensory examination should include analysis of large myelinated fibers (i.e., testing proprioception, vibratory sense, and in ambulatory ward patients, a Romberg test) and small fibers (i.e., pain and temperature sensation). Sensory complaints are characteristic of diseases affecting the sensory axons of peripheral nerves, plexus, or nerve roots. Isolated large fiber sensory loss may suggest a lesion in the dorsal columns (e.g., subacute combined degeneration in vitamin B12 deficiency).

Coordination should be analyzed with the patient's eyes open and closed to look for sensory or cerebellar ataxia.

Gait and posture testing where possible in ward patients should be observed for lordosis (i.e., stiff-person syndrome), a waddling gait (i.e., with myopathies), and a steppage gait (i.e., with polyneuropathies). The inability to rise from the floor or a chair suggests hip extensor weakness, whereas the inability to step up or down from a stool is consistent with a hip flexor or quadriceps muscle weakness. Clearly, these are not testable in most ICU consults.

Electrophysiologic tests (i.e., nerve conduction studies, electromyography, and repetitive stimulation tests) are valuable in diagnosing neuromuscular diseases (Case 45). Electromyography (EMG) can establish a peripheral nervous system disorder versus a central nervous system process (i.e., myelopathy) or psychogenic cause. It may also help differentiate among various peripheral nervous system disorders mentioned above. In addition to localizing the anatomy of the abnormality, EMG may provide information that will further narrow the differential diagnosis to a specific disease. Note that the time of onset of EMG/nerve conductien velocities (NCV) changes will depend on the distance and time needed for axonal degeneration to spread from the lesion to the muscle under study. This typically requires 10–21 days for fibrillations and positive waves to appear in the denervated muscle. For example, EMG and nerve conduction studies may help differentiate a neuropathic process into a demyelinating, axonal, sensory, or a motor neuropathy, thus minimizing ancillary investigations to the relevant diagnostic or confirmatory tests. On some occasions, electrophysiological testing can establish and follow the time course of disease progression or regression and be used to follow the effects of treatment.

43. Causes of paralysis and respiratory failure in the ICU

1. Myelopathies
2. ALS and other motor neuron disorders
3. Guillain-Barré syndrome
4. Toxic and vasculitic neuropathies
5. Chronic inflammatory demyelinating polyneuropathy
6. Porphyria
7. Myasthenia gravis and, rarely, Lambert-Eaton myasthenic syndrome and other myasthenic disorders
8. Tick paralysis
9. Botulism
10. Organophosphate poisoning
11. Prolonged neuromuscular junction blockade
12. Periodic paralysis
13. Critical illness neuromyopathy
14. Inflammatory myopathy
15. Toxic myopathy and other causes of rhabdomyolysis
16. Acid maltase myopathy
17. Muscular dystrophies, congenital myopathy, mitochondrial myopathy
18. Endocrine and electrolyte imbalance

Clinical Electrophysiology. By © Peter W. Kaplan and Thien Nguyen.
Published 2011 Blackwell Publishing Ltd.

44. The clinical evaluation of neuromuscular disorders

Characteristic	Myelopathy	Motor neuron disease	Polyneuropathy	Diseases of neuromuscular junction	Myopathy
Bulbar function	Normal	Opthalmoplegia, dysarthria, dysphagia in MG	Usually normal, but may be involve in Guillain-Barré syndrome	Dysarthria, dysphagia, and tongue weakness	Often normal, but may involve myositis and certain inherited myopathies
Pattern of weakness	Variable, usually symmetric	Variable, symmetric in most, but often asymmetric in ALS	Distal > proximal	Proximal > distal, fluctuates, often involves extraocular muscles	Proximal > distal
Muscle tone	Increased	Increased, but occasionally decreased	Decreased	Normal	Normal
Fasciculations	Normal, but sometimes in spondylotic myelopathy	Yes	Sometimes	No	No
Deep tendon reflexes	Increased	Variable, decreased in most, increased in ALS	Decreased or absent	Normal in postsynaptic (myasthenia gravis), decreased in presynaptic disorders (Lambert-Eaton syndrome and botulism)	Normal initially, may be decreased in later stage with severe weakness (ankle reflexes are often preserved until very late)
Babinski's sign	Upgoing toes	Upgoing toes	Normal	Normal	Normal
Sensory loss	Yes, often sensory level	No, except in Kennedy's disease	Usually present	No	No
Pain	Back pain	No	Often	No	Variable, usually no
Bowel/bladder dysfunction	Yes	No	No	No	No

Clinical Electrophysiology. By © Peter W. Kaplan and Thien Nguyen.
Published 2011 Blackwell Publishing Ltd.

45. Laboratory evaluation of neuromuscular disorders

Test	Motor neuron disease	Polyneuropathy	Diseases of neuromuscular junction	Myopathy
Serum creatine kinase (CK) level	May be mildly elevated	Normal	Normal	Increased
Nerve conduction studies	Normal or low-amplitude compound muscle action potential (CMAPs), normal sensory nerve action potential (SNAPs)	Slow nerve conduction velocities or low-amplitude Compound muscle action potential (CMAPs) and sensory nerve action potentials (SNAPs)	Normal	Normal
Electromyography	Decreased number of motor units (reduced recruitment), acute or chronic denervation/re-innervation	Decreased number of motor units (reduced recruitment), acute or chronic denervation/re-innervation	Normal, but may have voluntary motor units with small amplitude and short duration	Voluntary motor units with small amplitude and short duration
Repetitive nerve stimulation	Usually normal, but small decremental responses may occur	Normal	Decrement of CMAP at low rates of stimulation, large increment at fast rates in presynaptic disorders (30–100% in Botulism; >200% in Lambert-Eaton myasthenic syndrome (LEMS)); normal at fast rates in presynaptic disorders (normal or <25% in MG)	Normal
Muscle biopsy	Neurogenic denervation, fiber-type grouping, group atrophy	Neurogenic denervation, fiber-type grouping	Normal	Myopathic changes

Clinical Electrophysiology. By © Peter W. Kaplan and Thien Nguyen.
Published 2011 Blackwell Publishing Ltd.

Section B: Segmental weakness and/or sensory loss

Segmental weakness and sensory loss are common complaints in neuromuscular disorders in the ward. Attempts should be made to characterize the pattern of weakness: generalized, asymmetric, multifocal, proximally, distally, or lower versus upper extremity (Case 46).

Certain patterns of muscle weakness point to a peripheral nerve, plexus, or root lesion. With peripheral nerve causes, all muscles distal to the level of the lesion are vulnerable, but they are not necessarily equally affected. When multiple limb muscles are weak, localization depends on recognizing the common innervating nerve. A focal neuropathy (i.e., radial nerve palsy) or spinal nerve root lesion causes weakness limited to the distribution of the involved nerve or root. A complete plexopathy, such as traumatic brachial plexopathy, may cause weakness of the entire limb. However, a partial lesion may cause weakness only in the distribution of the affected plexus components. With some neuropathies, reflexes are typically decreased, often with sensory loss in the affected area. Anterior horn cell diseases often begin with focal weakness resembling a mononeuropathy, but will develop into a more widespread pattern as the disease progresses, culminating in generalized weakness. With the exception of extraocular muscle involvement in myasthenia gravis, it is rare for neuromuscular junction disorders or myopathies to cause focal weakness.

Electrophysiologic tests (i.e., nerve conduction studies, electromyography, and repetitive stimulation tests) are particularly valuable in localizing focal and segmental disorders, such as radiculopathies and nerve entrapment. These should be used to supplement the history and examination.

46. Evaluation of segmental peripheral neurological disorders

Characteristic	Mononeuropathy	Plexopathy	Radiculopathy
Pattern of weakness	Weakness in muscles innervated by a single nerve	Weakness in muscles innervated by different roots and nerves	Weakness in muscles innervated by the same root, but by different nerves
Reflex	Decreased reflexes in muscles innervated by a single nerve	Decreased in muscles innervated by roots from affected plexus, but by different nerves	Decreased in muscles innervated by the same root, but by different nerves
Sensory	Follows a single nerve territory	Follows patchy distribution of multiple roots and nerves	Follows the territory of the involved roots
Electromyography	Denervation in muscles innervated by a single nerve; normal paraspinous muscles	Denervation in muscles innervated by multiple roots and nerves; normal paraspinous muscles	Denervation in muscles innervated by the same root, but by different nerves; denervation in the affected paraspinous muscles
Sensory-evoked responses	Low-amplitude and/or prolonged SNAP latency	Low-amplitude SNAP in nerves from the affected plexus	Normal SNAPs
Motor nerve studies	Slow in affected nerve; low-amplitude CMAP or conduction block could be seen	Normal or low-amplitude CMAP in nerves from the affected plexus	Normal or low-amplitude CMAP in nerves from the affected plexus
Proximal responses (F-waves, H-reflexes)	Slow or absent in affected nerves	Slow or absent in nerves from the affected plexus	Slow or absent in nerves from affected roots

Clinical Electrophysiology. By © Peter W. Kaplan and Thien Nguyen.
Published 2011 Blackwell Publishing Ltd.

Section C: **Respiratory failure/diffuse weakness**

47. Amyotrophic lateral sclerosis/motor neuropathy

CLINICAL CORRELATES: Slowly progressive limb weakness over weeks to months, hyperreflexia, dysphagia, fasciculation, respiratory symptoms, and intact sensations.

ETIOLOGY: Motor neuronopathy.

CLINICAL EVALUATION: Look for slowly progressive limb weakness that may be asymmetrical: dysphagia, fasciculation, atrophy, and pathologic hyperreflexia. Body and limb sensations are normal.

ANCILLARY TESTING: Complete blood count, electrolytes including calcium and phosphate, liver function tests, thyroid studies, creatine kinase, erythrocyte sedimentation rate, anti-nuclear antibody, rheumatoid factor, vitamin B12, anti-GM1 antibody, serum protein electrophoresis with immunofixation, and 24-hour urine protein electrophoresis with immunofixation. Brain MRI whenever bulbar disease is present. Cervical and lumbosacral spine MRI to evaluate lower motor neuron (LMN) disease in the arms and legs. Normal cerebrospinal fluid (CSF). Screening for heavy metals in the blood and urine if there is known occupational exposure. Lumbar puncture and CSF analysis when there is clinical suspicion for Lyme disease, HIV infection, chronic inflammatory demyelinating polyneuropathy, or neoplasm. Sensory and motor nerve conduction studies and electromyography (EMG) are a standard part of the evaluation of motor neuron disease [1].

DIFFERENTIAL DIAGNOSIS: Asymmetrical weakness suggests inflammatory myopathy, neuromuscular junction disorders (i.e., myasthenia gravis), thyrotoxicosis, acute polyneuropathies, cervical spondylosis with nerve root compression, multifocal motor neuropathy (MMN), and motor neuron diseases. Myopathies do not have these EMG findings, asymmetrical weakness, and hyperreflexia. Myasthenia gravis (MG) may clinically comprise dysarthria, dysphagia, and limb and facial weakness without ptosis or ocular dysmotility, and thus mimic bulbar amyotrophic lateral sclerosis (ALS). Upper motor neuron (UMN) or LMN bulbar signs, absence of ocular findings, and lack of diurnal variation of symptoms argue against MG. Thyrotoxicosis may include UMN signs related to pyramidal tract dysfunction and LMN signs related to a peripheral neuropathy and mimic ALS. MMN, also known as MMN with conduction block, is characterized by LMN signs often with a bibrachial pattern. Motor nerve conduction studies in MMN usually often shows conduction block (focal demyelination). Sensory conduction is normal. Raised GM1 antibodies occur in 30–80% of patients with MMN. UMN signs, diffuse acute or chronic denervations, and the absence of conduction block would argue against MMN. Lack of history of polio argues against this cause. The clinical hallmark of a selective motor deficit, the combination of UMN and LMN signs, asymmetrical weakness, bulbar involvement, and an EMG showing acute or chronic denervation/re-innervation in three or more segments point toward ALS [2, 3].

PROGNOSIS: ALS is a progressive neurodegenerative disorder that causes muscle weakness, disability, and eventually death, with a median survival of 3–5 years [4]. While the rate of progression between individuals is variable, the history should reflect gradual and progressive worsening over time without intervening remissions or exacerbations. The progressive course of ALS eventually produces one or both of the life-threatening aspects of the disease, neuromuscular respiratory failure, and dysphagia.

TREATMENT: There is no cure for ALS. Expert consensus guideline recommendations by the American Academy of Neurology [5] cover breaking the news of the

Clinical Electrophysiology. By © Peter W. Kaplan and Thien Nguyen. Published 2011 Blackwell Publishing Ltd.

Motor nerve conduction

Nerve and site	Latency	Amplitude	Distance	Conduction velocity
Peroneal.R				
Ankle	5.4 ms	1.2 mV	mm	m/s
Fibula (head)	0.7 ms	1.0 mV	240 mm	45 m/s
Popliteal fossa	12.5 ms	1.0 mV	90 mm	50 m/s
Tibial.R				
Ankle	6.1 ms	1.0 mV	mm	m/s
Tibial.L				
Ankle	5.4 ms	1.2 mV	mm	m/s
Peroneal.L				
Fibula (head)	3.0 ms	2.1 mV	mm	m/s
Popliteal fossa	4.6 ms	2.6 mV	90 mm	56 m/s
Median.R				
Wrist	NR ms	mV	mm	m/s
Ulnar.R				
Wrist	NR ms	mV	mm	m/s

Sensory nerve conduction

Nerve and site	Peak latency	Amplitude	Segment	Latency difference	Distance	Conduction velocity
Sural.R						
Point B	3.2 ms	14 µV	Lateral malleolus-Point B	2.2 ms	105 mm	48 m/s
Median.R						
Wrist	4.1 ms	11 µV	Digit II (index finger)-Wrist	2.5 ms	130 mm	52 m/s
Ulnar.R						
Wrist	3.1 ms	17 µV	Digit V (little finger)-Wrist	2.1 ms	110 mm	50 m/s

diagnosis, nutrition, respiratory management, palliative care, and the use of riluzole. Respiratory management and nutrition are important symptomatic issues facing patients with ALS. Symptomatic management is the mainstay of treatment for ALS. Therapy should be offered in a multidisciplinary environment where physical therapists, occupational therapists, and speech therapists can assist with the management of dysarthria, dysphagia, activities of daily living, and functional decline. Patients treated by multidisciplinary ALS centers have improved survival compared with those followed by general neurology clinics. Only riluzole has been approved by the Food and Drug Administration for extending survival in ALS. Patients most likely to benefit from riluzole include (1) ALS by El-Escorial criteria, (2) symptoms present for less than 5 years, (3) vital capacity greater than 60% of predicted, and (4) no tracheostomy.

NCV: These sensory nerve action potentials are normal; right median and ulnar motor responses are absent. Both tibial and right peroneal CMAP amplitudes are reduced. Concentric needle EMG examination shows diffuse acute denervation (i.e., fibrillations and positive sharp waves). There are reduced or neurogenic recruitment and voluntary motor units with long duration and large amplitude. Many motor units are polyphasic.

In general, the abnormalities are most marked in the weak limbs, but may occur in asymptomatic limbs. Fasciculation potentials may be seen in asymptomatic limbs.

In summary, acute or chronic denervation/re-innervation involving ventral nerve roots or spinal cord segments. These findings are consistent with an active polyradiculopathy (such as carcinomatous meningitis), a diffuse myelopathy, or progressive motor neuron disease. The absence of radicular pain and sensory deficit suggests ALS.

REFERENCES:

1. Daube JR. Electrodiagnostic studies in amyotrophic lateral sclerosis and other motor neuron disorders. *Muscle Nerve* 2000;23:1488.

2. Brooks BR. El Escorial world federation of neurology criteria for the diagnosis of amyotrophic lateral sclerosis. Subcommittee on motor neuron diseases/amyotrophic lateral sclerosis of the World Federation of Neurology Research Group on neuromuscular diseases and the El Escorial clinical limits of amyotrophic lateral sclerosis workshop contributors. *J Neurol Sci* 1994;124(Suppl):96.

3. Brooks BR, Miller RG, Swash M, Munsat TL; World Federation of Neurology Research Group on Motr Neuron Diseases. El Escorial revisited: Revised criteria for the diagnosis of amyotrophic lateral sclerosis. *Amyotroph Lateral Scler Other Motor Neuron Disord* 2000;1:293.

4. Mitsumoto H, Chad DA, Pioro EP. Amyotrophic lateral sclerosis. *Contemporary Neurology Series*, volume 49, Philadelphia, PA: FA Davis 1998;480.

5. Miller RG, Rosenberg JA, Gelinas DF, Mitsumoto H, Newman D, Sufit R, Borasio GD, Bradley WG, Bromberg MB, Brooks BR, Kassrkis EJ, Munsat TL, Oppenheimer EA. Practice parameter: the care of the patient with amyotrophic lateral sclerosis (an evidence-based review): Report of the quality standards subcommittee of the American Academy of Neurology: ALS Practice Parameters Task Force. *Neurology* 1999;52:1311.

48. Critical illness neuromyopathy

CLINICAL CORRELATES: Diffuse limb weakness, impaired sensation, and hyporeflexia. Failure to wean off ventilator.

ETIOLOGY: Neuropathy.

CLINICAL EVALUATION: For critical illness polyneuropathy/myopathy, look for [1] setting of critical illness such as sepsis, multiorgan failure, and the systemic inflammatory response syndrome [2], difficulty weaning from ventilator not related to cardiopulmonary causes [3], exposure to paralytic and/or steroids [4], and limb weakness (usually the legs). Patients show facial expression to pain even while the limbs cannot withdraw. There is relative sparing of cranial nerves, depressed or absent reflexes and electrophysiologic evidence of axonal motor and sensory polyneuropathy, or irritable myopathy.

ANCILLARY TESTING: Complete blood count, electrolytes including calcium and phosphate, liver function tests, thyroid studies, creatine kinase, erythrocyte sedimentation rate, anti-nuclear antibody, rheumatoid factor, vitamin B12, serum protein electrophoresis with immunofixation, and 24-hour urine protein electrophoresis with immunofixation. Brain MRI whenever bulbar disease is present. Cervical and lumbosacral spine MRI to evaluate lower motor neuron disease in the arms and legs. Anti-AChR and anti-MuSk antibodies. Rule out other neuropathic process including Guillain-Barré syndrome, porphyria, and heavy metal intoxication. Sensory and motor nerve conduction studies and electromyography (EMG) are a standard part of the evaluation of critical illness polyneuropathy.

DIFFERENTIAL DIAGNOSIS: See Table 48.1. Neuromuscular transmission disorders manifest with ptosis, unrespon-

Table 48.1 Causes of paralysis and respiratory failure in ICU

1. Myelopathies
2. ALS and othe motor neuron disorders
3. Myasthenia gravis and rarely, Lambert-Eaton myasthic syndrome an other myasthenic
4. Tick paralysis
5. Botulism
6. Organophosphate poisoning
7. Prolonged neuromuscular junction blockade
8. Guillain-Barre syndrome
9. Toxic and vasculitic neuropathies
10. Chronic inflammatory demyelinating polyneuropathy
11. Porphyria
12. Critical illness neuromyopathy
13. Inflammatory myopathy
14. Toxic myopathy and other causes of rhabdomyolysis
15. Acid maltase myopathy
16. Muscular dystrophies, congenital myopathy, mitochondrial myopathy
17. Endocrine and electrolyte imbalance

sive pupils, or ophthalmoplegia. Review of the patient's drug list will help to eliminate the possibility of toxic myopathy or even exogenous toxins (organophosphates). The diagnosis is critical illness neuromyopathy. A muscle biopsy with myosin loss would be helpful in confirming the diagnosis.

PROGNOSIS: Mortality is approximately 26–71% dependent on the severity of the underlying primary disease [3]. Recovery can take months, with up to 50% of the patients having complete recovery; many have persistent functional disability with reduced quality of life. Electrodiagnostic testing may demonstrate residual nerve dysfunction several years after initial presentation [4].

TREATMENT: No specific therapy. Weaning of steroids is recommended. Supportive management and

Clinical Electrophysiology. By © Peter W. Kaplan and Thien Nguyen. Published 2011 Blackwell Publishing Ltd.

Sensory nerve conduction

Nerve and site	Peak latency	Amplitude	Segment	Latency difference	Distance	Conduction velocity
Sural.L						
Point B	3.5 ms	4 µV	Lateral malleolus-Point B	2.5 ms	100 mm	40 m/s
Sural.R						
Point B	NR ms	µV	Lateral malleolus-Point B	ms	mm	m/s
Median.L						
Digit II	NR ms	µV	Wrist-Digit II	ms	mm	m/s
Ulnar.L						
V Digit	NR ms	µV	Wrist-V Digit	ms	mm	m/s
Radial.L						
Forearm	NR ms	µV	Dorsum of hand-Forearm	ms	mm	m/s

Motor nerve conduction

Nerve and site	Latency	Amplitude	Distance	Conduction velocity
Peroneal.L				
Ankle	3.6 ms	1.4 mV	mm	m/s
Fibula (head)	14.2 ms	0.5 mV	250 mm	40 m/s
Popliteal fossa	16.5 ms	0.4 mV	100 mm	43 m/s
Tibial.L				
Ankle	4.7 ms	1.4 mV	mm	m/s
Tibial.R				
Ankle	4.4 ms	1.3 mV	mm	m/s
Peroneal.R				
Ankle	4.3 ms	1.9 mV	mm	m/s
Fibula (head)	13.2 ms	1.4 mV	290 mm	39 m/s
Popliteal fossa	15.2 ms	1.3 mV	80 mm	40 m/s
Median.L				
Wrist	3.2 ms	6.8 mV	mm	m/s
Antecubital	8.4 ms	4.9 mV	230 mm	49 m/s
Ulnar.L				
Wrist	3.1 ms	1.9 mV	mm	49 m/s

Needle EMG data

		Insertional				Activation				
		Ins Act	Fibs	+Wave	Fasc	Amplitude	Duration	Config	Rate	Activation
Deltoid Middle	R	Normal	1+	1+	None	SD	SD	Norm	None	EARLY
Biceps Brachii	R	Normal	None	1+	None	MD	MD	Norm	None	EARLY
Triceps Med H	R	Normal	None	None	None	MD	MD	Norm	None	EARLY
Gastroc Med Hd	R	Normal	None	None	None	Norm	Norm	Norm	None	Norm
Tibialis Ant	R	Normal	None	None	None	MD	MD	Norm	None	Norm
Tibialis Ant	L	Normal	None	None	None	Norm	Norm	Norm	None	Norm
Glut Med	L	Normal	None	None	None	SI	SI	Norm	None	Norm

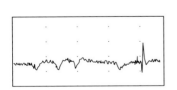

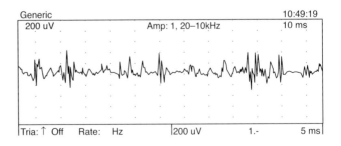

rehabilitation are required—intensive pulmonary hygiene and prevention of skin breakdown, contractures, and deep vein thrombosis, and superimposed compressive neuropathies. Long-term—physical rehabilitation, assistive devices, and pain medications.

NCVS: These show marked reduction of compound muscle action potential amplitudes, with relatively preservation of conduction velocities and latencies, decreased sensory nerve action potential amplitudes. With the asymmetric deficit, these suggest an acquired axonal polyneuropathy. It is a mixed motor and sensory neuropathy. Needle EMG may show fibrillation potentials and positive sharp waves (denervation) with normal motor units. EMG may show early recruitment, short duration, small amplitude voluntary motor units (myopathic changes). It is often clinically difficult to distinguish between critical illness polyneuropathy and critical illness myopathy—the two may occur together—"critical illness neuromyopathy" [1, 2].

REFERENCES:

1. Op de Coul AA, Verheul GA, Leyten AC, Schellens RL, Teepen JL. Critical illness polyneuromyopathy after artificial respiration. *Clin Neurol Neurosurg* 1991;93:27.
2. Bednarik J, Lukas Z, Vondracek P. Critical illness polyneuromyopathy: The electrophysiological components of a complex entity. *Intensive Care Med* 2003;29:1505.
3. Kane SL, Dasta JF. Clinical outcomes of critical illness polyneuropathy. *Pharmacotherapy* 2002;22(3):373–379.
4. Fletcher SN, Kennedy DD, Ghosh IR, Misra VP, Kiff K, Coakley JH, Hinds CJ. Persistent neuromuscular and neurophysiologic abnormalities in long-term survivors of prolonged critical illness. *Crit Care Med* 2003;31:1012.

49. Brachial plexopathy

ER, ward

CLINICAL CORRELATES: Acute arm pain, followed by progressive weakness, predominantly of the shoulder girdle muscles. Patchy numbness in the hand and forearm, worse in the thumb.

ETIOLOGY: Brachial plexopathy.

CLINICAL EVALUATION: Look for distribution of weakness, onset of symptoms, pain, sensory loss, and depressed or absent deep tendon reflexes supplied by the plexus.

ANCILLARY TESTING: Complete blood count (infection), creatine kinase, erythrocyte sedimentation rate, antinuclear antibody, rheumatoid factor, anti-GM1 antibody (for multifocal motor neuropathy), serum protein electrophoresis with immunofixation (lymphoma), and 24-hour urine protein electrophoresis with immunofixation (myeloma). Cervical spine and brachial plexus CT or MRI to look for structural problems. Nerve conduction studies and needle electromyography localize terminal segments of nerves and the distribution of abnormalities.

DIFFERENTIAL DIAGNOSIS: Frequent causes are trauma, neuralgic amyotrophy, hereditary brachial plexopathy, neoplastic and radiation-induced brachial plexopathy, thoracic outlet syndrome, diabetic-related brachial plexopathy, and iatrogenic plexopathies. The presence of sensory loss, diminished reflexes, and radiating pain represents peripheral nervous system disorders such radiculopathy, plexopathy, or neuropathy. The pattern of a sensory loss and weakness within a defined nerve root or nerve suggests a plexopathy. Acute onset, in the absence of trauma, favors a metabolic or inflammatory process. The absence of a chronic progression of symptoms, the presence of pain, and the absence of a history of cancer and radiation treatment argue against radiation associated plexopathy. This most likely represents idiopathic brachial plexitis or neuralgic amyotrophy.

PROGNOSIS: Long-term prognosis is good. Pain resolves within weeks. Improvement in muscle strength lags behind; most patients recover completely within a few months [1]. With marked axonal involvement/affected distal muscles, recovery can be protracted. Recurrence of idiopathic neuralgic amyotrophy was reported in 26%; median time to recurrence is approximately 2 years [2].

TREATMENT: No specific treatment. Glucocorticoids may help with pain [2], but may not affect outcome. Physical and occupational therapies help avoid contractures.

NCVs: The right median and lateral antebrachial cutaneous sensory responses are absent; right ulnar and medial antebrachial cutaneous SNAP amplitudes are reduced. The right radial SNAP amplitude is reduced; left ulnar, medial and lateral antebrachial cutaneous, median, and radial sensory responses are normal. The abnormal SNAPs indicate a plexopathy or multiple neuropathies (not a particular nerve or nerve root). The right median and axillary CMAP amplitudes are markedly reduced. These findings suggest a possible upper trunk lesion. Needle electromyography examination shows diffuse denervation in all muscles tested on the right except the paraspinous and rhomboid muscles. This points to a diffuse multifocal process involving all neural elements of the brachial plexus, with more severe involvement of the upper trunk of brachial plexus and the anterior interosseus nerve, consistent with neuralgic amyotrophy (or brachial plexopathy).

REFERENCES:
1. Tsairis P, Dyck PJ, Mulder DW. Natural history of brachial plexus neuropathy. Report on 99 patients. *Arch Neurol* 1972;27:109.
2. van Alfen N, van Engelen BG. The clinical spectrum of neuralgic amyotrophy in 246 cases. *Brain* 2006;129:438.

Sensory nerve conduction

Nerve and site	Peak latency	Amplitude	Segment	Latency difference	Distance	Conduction velocity
Ulnar.R						
Wrist	3.2 ms	4 µV	Digit V (little finger)-Wrist	2.6 ms	120 mm	47 m/s
Median.R						
Wrist	NR ms	µV	Digit II (index finger)-Wrist	ms	mm	m/s
Radial.R						
Forearm	1.9 ms	15 µV	Dorsum of hand-Forearm	1.3 ms	70 mm	54 m/s
Ulnar.L						
Wrist	3.1 ms	13 µV	Digit V (little finger)-Wrist	2.3 ms	120 mm	50 m/s
Median.L						
Wrist	4.1 ms	17 µV	Digit II (index finger)-Wrist	2.5 ms	130 mm	52 m/s
Radial.L						
Forearm	1.9 ms	27 µV	Dorsum of hand-Forearm	1.3 ms	70 mm	54 m/s
Lateral antebrachial cutaneous.R						
Elbow	NR ms	µV	Forearm-Elbow	14.7 ms	mm	m/s
Medial antebrachial cutaneous.R						
Elbow	2.5 ms	5 µV	Forearm-Elbow	2.0 ms	100 mm	50 m/s
Lateral antebrachial cutaneous.L						
Elbow	3.0 ms	17 µV	Forearm-Elbow	2.3 ms	115 mm	50 m/s
Medial antebrachial cutaneous.L						
Elbow	2.5 ms	20 µV	Forearm-Elbow	2.0 ms	110 mm	55 m/s

Motor nerve conduction

Nerve and site	Latency	Normal limits	Amplitude	Normal limits	Distance	Conduction velocity	Normal limits
Median.R							
Wrist	4.2 ms		0.5 mV		mm	m/s	
Antecubital	8.7 ms		0.4 mV		255 mm	57 m/s	
Ulnar.R							
Wrist	2.4 ms		5.7 mV		mm	m/s	
Below elbow	6.4 ms		3.3 mV		270 mm	64 m/s	
Above elbow	8.5 ms		2.8 mV		90 mm	50 m/s	
Axillary.R							
Erb's point	3.6 ms		0.4 mV		mm	m/s	
Median.L							
Wrist	4.0 ms		7.4 mV		mm	m/s	
Antecubital	8.5 ms		6.8 mV		250 mm	54 m/s	
Ulnar.L							
Wrist	2.3 ms		8.7 mV		mm	m/s	
Below elbow	6.2 ms		6.1 mV		265 mm	65 m/s	
Above elbow	8.4 ms		5.6 mV		85 mm	55 m/s	
Axillary.L							
Erb's point	3.3 ms		5.1 mV		mm	m/s	

Needle EMG examination

	Insertional	Spontaneous activity			Volitional MUAPs					
Muscle	Insertional	+ Wave	Fibs	Fasc	Activation	Rate	Duration	Amplitude	Config	Other
1st dorsal interosseous.R	Normal	None	None	None	None	Normal	Normal	Normal	Normal	Normal
Abductor pollicis brevis.R	Normal	None	None	None	None	Normal	Normal	Normal	Normal	Normal
Pronator teres.R	Normal	+1	+1	None	None	Reduced	Normal	Normal	Normal	Normal
Flex. digit. prof.R	Normal	+2	+2	None	None	Reduced	Normal	Normal	Normal	Normal
Brachioradialis.R	Normal	+2	+2	None	no units					
Triceps.R	Normal	+1	+1	None	None	Reduced	Normal	Normal	Normal	Normal
Biceps.R	Normal	+2	+2	None	no units					
Deltoid.R	Normal	+2	+2	None	no units					
C-5 Paraspinous.R	Normal	None	None	None	None	Normal	Normal	Normal	Normal	Normal
Infraspinatus.R	Normal	+2	+2	None	no units					
Rhomboid minor.R	Normal	None	None	None	None	Normal	Normal	Normal	Normal	Normal
Supraspinatus.R	Normal	+2	+2	None	no units					

50. Femoral neuropathy

CLINICAL CORRELATES: Severe leg weakness, numbness in the anterior thigh and leg, and inability to walk after pelvic surgery. Patellar reflexes absent.

ETIOLOGY: Femoral neuropathy secondary to pelvic surgery, direct trauma, compression, stretch injury, ischemia, and diabetes.

CLINICAL EVALUATION: Weakness of the quadriceps muscle and a decreased patellar reflex. Wasting of the quadriceps in advanced and chronic cases. When the iliopsoas muscle is involved, the lesion is above the inguinal ligament. In isolated femoral neuropathies, the thigh adductors are normal (innervated by the obturator nerve). Sensory deficits—numbness of the medial thigh and the anteromedial calf. Pain with hip extension with a retroperitoneal hematoma.

ANCILLARY TESTING: Complete blood count (drop after hematoma). CT for hematoma, MRI to detect bony abnormalities. Nerve conduction studies and needle electromyography (EMG) localize terminal segments of nerves and the distribution of abnormalities.

DIFFERENTIAL DIAGNOSIS: The history of pelvic surgery excludes the more indolent and most other neuropathies. The presence of sensory loss and diminished patellar reflexes is consistent with peripheral nervous system disorder such radiculopathy, plexopathy, or neuropathy. The weakness and sensory loss are limited to muscles and area innervated by the femoral nerve. Likewise, the EMG localizes the lesion to the femoral nerve. The involvement of the iliopsoas muscle suggests an intrapelvic compressive femoral neuropathy.

Clinical Electrophysiology. By © Peter W. Kaplan and Thien Nguyen. Published 2011 Blackwell Publishing Ltd.

PROGNOSIS: Recovery is good and typically occurs over 3–6 months [1].

TREATMENT: With a retroperitoneal hematoma, evacuation of the hematoma is occasionally done, but usually not. If possible, anticoagulant agents should be stopped until the hematoma has resolved. Outcomes for these patients are worse than for those with a hematoma due to trauma. If the compression is due to a tumor, then therapy, either surgery or chemotherapy, is directed at the neoplasm. Possible surgical decompression is done for mass lesions. With vasculitic causes, immunosuppressive therapy may help. Management comprises intensive physiotherapy [2] and knee bracing. Some clinicians suggest surgical exploration when symptoms fail to improve in 14 weeks [3,4].

NCVs: These show an absent right saphenous sensory nerve action potential (SNAP) and a normal left saphenous SNAP (which excludes an L4 root lesion). There are normal and symmetric femoral motor studies. Wallerian's degeneration may take up 10 days for axonal degeneration to complete. Needle EMG shows acute denervation in the right quadriceps and iliopsoas muscles, but it is normal in the thigh adductors and anterior tibialis muscles. Normal thigh adductors would exclude a lumbar plexopathy. Involvement of the iliopsoas muscles suggests an intrapelvic femoral nerve lesion occurring from compression of retractor compression against the pelvic wall during pelvic surgery and is not a compression of the femoral nerve at the inguinal ligament, such as occurs during lithotomy positioning. Evaluation for a femoral nerve dysfunction includes nerve conduction studies (NCS) and needle EMG. NCS should include sensory studies of the saphenous nerve and motor studies of the femoral nerve. When evaluating femoral NCS, results on the symptomatic side should be compared to those on the asymptomatic side. On EMG, the quadriceps should show neuropathic changes. The iliopsoas is involved if

Sensory nerve conduction

Nerve and site	Peak latency	Amplitude	Segment	Latency difference	Distance	Conduction velocity
Sural.R						
Point B	3.2 ms	14 µV	Lateral malleolus-Point B	2.2 ms	105 mm	48 m/s
Saphenous.R						
Media Tibia	2.8 ms	4 µV	Medial Malleolus-Medial Tibia	2.8 ms	110 mm	m/s
Saphenous.L						
Media Tibia	NR ms	µV	Medial Malleolus-Medial Tibia	ms	mm	0 m/s

Motor nerve conduction

Nerve and site	Latency	Amplitude	Distance	Conduction velocity
Peroneal.L				
Ankle	3.6 ms	1.4 mV	mm	m/s
Fibula (head)	14.2 ms	1.5 mV	250 mm	40 m/s
Popliteal fossa	16.5 ms	1.4 mV	100 mm	43 m/s
Tibial.L				
Ankle	4.7 ms	1.4 mV	mm	m/s
Tibial.R				
Ankle	4.4 ms	1.3 mV	mm	m/s
Peroneal.R				
Ankle	4.3 ms	1.9 mV	mm	m/s
Fibula (head)	13.2 ms	1.4 mV	290 mm	39 m/s
Popliteal fossa	15.2 ms	1.3 mV	80 mm	40 m/s
Femoral.R				
Groin	6.1 ms	3.1 mV	mm	m/s
Femoral.L				
Groin	5.7 ms	5.6 mV	mm	m/s

Needle EMG examination

Muscle	Insertional	Spontaneous activity			Volitional MUAPs					
	Insertional	+ Wave	Fibs	Fasc	Activation	Rate	Duration	Amplitude	Config	Other
Vastus lateralis.R	Increased	+3	+3	None	GD	Rapid	Normal	Normal	Normal	
Rectus femoris.R	Increased	+2	+2	None	GD	Rapid	Normal	Normal	Normal	
Iliopsoas.R	Increased	+2	+2	None	MD	Normal	SI	SI	Polyphasic	
Thigh adductor.R	Normal	None	None	None	Normal	Normal	Normal	Normal	Normal	
Med gastrocnemius.R	Normal	None	None	None	Normal	Normal	Normal	Normal	Normal	
Gluteus medius.R	Normal	None	None	None	Normal	Normal	Normal	Normal	Normal	
L5-paraspinous.R	Normal	None	None	None	Normal	Normal	Normal	Normal	Normal	
Vastus lateralis.R	Normal	None	None	None	Normal	Normal	Normal	Normal	Normal	

the lesion is in the pelvis (above the inguinal ligament). The adductor magnus and brevis, which share lumbar innervation with quadriceps and iliopsoas, are spared (innervated primarily by the obturator and sciatic nerves).

REFERENCES:

1. Goldman JA, Feldberg D, Dicker D. Femoral neuropathy subsequent to abdominal hysterectomy: A comprehensive study. *Eur J Obstet Gynecol Reprod Biol* 1985;20:385–392.

2. Celebrezze JP Jr, Pidala MJ, Porter JA, Slezak FA. Femoral neuropathy: An infrequently reported postoperative complication. Report of four cases. *Dis Colon Rectum* 2000;43:419–422.

3. Georgy FM. Femoral neuropathy following abdominal hysterectomy. *Am J Obstet Gynecol* 1975;123:819–822.

4. Brasch RC, Bufo AJ, Kreienberg PF, Johnson GP. Femoral neuropathy secondary to the use of a self-retaining retractor. Report of three cases and review of the literature. *Dis Colon Rectum* 1995;38:1115–1118.

51. Sensory neuropathy/ganglionopathy [1–3]

ER, MICU, WARD

CLINICAL CORRELATES: Progressive dysphagia, weight loss, and facial dysesthesias. No weakness, dry eyes and mouth. There is marked loss of large and small fiber sensory modalities in a length-dependent fashion, hyporeflexia, and ataxic gait.

ETIOLOGY: Sensory neuropathy or ganglionopathy.

CLINICAL EVALUATION: Look for a specific pattern of joint, muscle, and sensory loss in a non-length-dependent pattern, leading to distinct clinical, neurophysiological, and neuropathological findings. Normal strength and sensory ataxia.

ANCILLARY TESTING: Liver function tests (hepatitis), erythrocyte sedimentation rate, anti-nuclear antibody, rheumatoid factor, paraneoplastic panel, serum protein electrophoresis with immunofixation, 24-hour urine protein electrophoresis with immunofixation, anti-Ro, anti-La, anti-Sm, and anti-ribonucleoprotein antibodies. Obtain cerebrospinal fluid (CSF) to evaluate for inflammation (including elevated CSF protein and mononuclear cells) and infection (i.e., Lyme disease, syphilis, and cytomegalovirus). Consider skin biopsy for pattern of sensory fiber loss.

DIFFERENTIAL DIAGNOSIS: Autoimmune (i.e., paraneoplastic ganglionopathy, paraproteinemia, or polyclonal gammopathy), drugs (thalidomide, pyridoxine, *cis*-platinum, doxorubicin, etc.), inflammatory (Sjögren's syndrome, acute sensory polyneuropathy, chronic inflmatory sensory polyneuropathy, etc.), hereditary (hereditary sensory axonal neuropathy, Fabry's disease, Friedreich's ataxia, spinocerebellar degeneration), infections (i.e., syphilis, Lyme, and herpes zoster), and idiopathic ganglionoapthy. Inherited ganglionopathy usually manifests a slow progression and positive family history. Look for possible neurotoxic drugs: thalidomide, *cis*-platinum [1], high-dose pyridoxine. Focal sensory

ganglionitis may occur in viral or bacterial infections (herpes zoster and, possibly, *Borrelia burgdorferi*). Sensory neuronopathy occurs with inflammatory or autoimmune diseases, ataxic neuronopathy (with Sjögren's syndrome). Sjögren's syndrome includes dry eyes and mouth (sicca syndrome); articular symptoms, inflammatory arthropathy, or occasionally rheumatoid arthritis [1]. These with gait impairment and proprioception loss suggest Sjögren's syndrome sensory neuronopathy

PROGNOSIS: It depends on the etiology, but it is generally poor. In Sjögren's syndrome, progression is usually slow and insidious. Symptoms will often be stable over many years.

TREATMENT: There is no definitive treatment [2]. Treatment is focused on symptomatic pain relief. There has been poor response to most immunotherapy.

NCVS: The motor system is spared clinically and electrophysiologically. There is a widespread decrease in sensory nerve action potential (SNAP) amplitudes, with no proximal–distal gradient. The amplitude of SNAPs in the upper limbs is lower than in the lower limbs. The non-length-dependent distribution of sensory loss in a manner suggests a dorsal root ganglionopathy, often called a sensory neuronopathy or ganglionopathy [1].

REFERENCES:
1. Govoni M, Bajocchi G, Rizzo N, Tola MR, Caniatti L, Tugnoli V, Colamussi P, Trotta F. Neurological involvement in primary Sjögren's syndrome: Clinical and instrumental evaluation in a cohort of Italian patients. *Clin Rheumatol* 1999;18(4):299–303.
2. Venables PJ. Sjögren's syndrome. *Best Pract Res Clin Rheumatol* 2004;18:313–329.
3. Jonsson R, Haga HJ, Gordon T. Sjögren's syndrome. In: Koopman WJ (ed.), *Arthritis and Allied Conditions: A Textbook of Rheumatology*, 14th edn. Philadelphia, PA: Lippincott Williams & Wilkins 2001:1736–1759.

Sensory nerve conduction

Nerve and site	Peak latency	Amplitude	Segment	Latency difference	Distance	Conduction velocity
Sural.L						
Point B	3.5 ms	4 μV	Lateral malleolus-Point B	2.5 ms	100 mm	40 m/s
Sural.R						
Point B	3.5 ms	4 μV	Lateral malleolus-Point B	2.5 ms	100 mm	40 m/s
Median.L						
Digit II	NR ms	μV	Wrist-Digit II	ms	mm	m/s
Ulnar.L						
V Digit	NR ms	μV	Wrist-V Digit	ms	mm	m/s
Radial.L						
Forearm	NR ms	μV	Dorsum of hand-Forearm	ms	mm	m/s

Motor nerve conduction

Nerve and site	Latency	Amplitude	Segment	Latency difference	Distance	Conduction velocity
Peroneal.R						
Ankle	5.4 ms	6.7 mV	EDB-Ankle	5.4 ms	mm	m/s
Fibular Head	13.2 ms	6.0 mV	Ankle-Fibular Head	7.8 ms	310 mm	40 m/s
Pop Fossa	15.2 ms	5.7 mV	Fibular Head-Pop Fossa	2.0 ms	90 mm	45 m/s
Tibial.R						
ankle	4.7 ms	14.5 mV	AH-ankle	4.7 ms	mm	m/s
Tibial.L						
ankle	4.6 ms	16.9 mV	AH-ankle	4.6 ms	mm	m/s
Peroneal.L						
Ankle	5.3 ms	4.3 mV	EDB-Ankle	5.3 ms	mm	m/s
Fibular Head	12.8 ms	4.3 mV	Ankle-Fibular Head	7.5 ms	310 mm	41 m/s
Pop fossa	14.2 ms	3.8 mV	Fibular Head-Pop Fossa	1.4 ms	100 mm	71 m/s
Median.L						
wrist	3.0 ms	4.4 mV	APB-wrist	3.0 ms	mm	m/s
antecubital	7.6 ms	3.4 mV	wrist-antecubital	4.6 ms	250 mm	54 m/s
Ulnar.L						
wrist	3.0 ms	3.8 mV	wrist	3.0 ms	mm	m/s

Needle EMG examination

Muscle	Insertional	Spontaneous activity			Volitional MUAPs					
	Insertional	+ Wave	Fibs	Fasc	Activation	Rate	Duration	Amplitude	Config	Other
Iliopsoas.L	Normal	None	None	None	None	Normal	Normal	Normal	Normal	Normal
Rectus femoris.L	Normal	None	None	None	None	Normal	Normal	Normal	Normal	Normal
Tibialis anterior.L	Normal	None	None	None	None	Normal	Normal	Normal	Normal	Normal
Gastrocnemius (Medial head).L	Normal	None	None	None	None	Normal	Normal	Normal	Normal	Normal

F-wave studies

Nurve	M-Latency	F-Latency
Peroneal.L	5.5	61.7
Tibial.L	5.3	61.5
Tibial.R	4.5	56.8
Peroneal.R	4.4	59.9
Median.L	3.4	30.1

52. Lumbar radiculopathy [1–3]

ER, MICU

CLINICAL CORRELATES: Pain radiating down the right buttock to the lateral thigh and pretibial area, worse with ambulation. Right foot weakness with footdrop; frequent tripping and falls. Gait difficulty.

ETIOLOGY: Lumbar radiculopathy or neuropathy.

CLINICAL EVALUATION: Look for pain in a dermatomal distribution (radicular pain), sensory loss and weakness in corresponding dermatomal distribution, and absent or depressed reflexes. Sitting, coughing, or sneezing may exacerbate the pain. Often, an assessment of the L5 reflex (medial hamstrings) is helpful. Provocative maneuvers, such as the straight-leg raising test, may provide evidence of increased dural tension, indicating underlying nerve root pathology.

ANCILLARY TESTING: Erythrocyte sedimentation rate, anti-nuclear antibody, and rheumatoid factor. Consider a lumbar spine MRI to detect bony abnormalities, disc herniation, nerve root compression, and structural abnormalities. Nerve conduction studies and needle electromyography (EMG) localize terminal segments of nerves and the distribution of abnormalities.

DIFFERENTIAL DIAGNOSIS: Myelopathy, radiculopathy, plexopathy, single or multiple neuropathy, demyelinating conditions, and spondylolysis. Sensory loss and diminished reflexes suggest a peripheral nervous system process. Pain radiation in the buttock to the lateral thigh and leg suggests an L5 dermatomal distribution (cf. the distribution of sensory impairment in the lateral leg and dorsum of the foot). Weakness of ankle and toe dorsiflexion represents an L5 nerve root process. However, absent ankle reflexes and ankle plantar flexion weakness

suggest possible superimposed involvement of the S1 radiculopathy. A plexopathy or sciatic neuropathy cannot be excluded. EMG confirms an L5–S1 nerve root lesion by involvement of muscles outside sciatic nerve distribution and proximal to the lumbosacral plexus (i.e., paraspinous muscles). To differentiate between an L3 radiculopathy and a femoral neuropathy, weakness in the hip adductors in addition to the quadriceps group indicates an L3 radiculopathy. With isolated femoral neuropathy, only the quadriceps group would be weak.

PROGNOSIS: It depends on the cause. Most radiculopathies arise from nerve root compression by lumbar spondylosis or disc herniation, and prognosis is excellent with medical treatment (80–90% of patients can be treated medically) [1,2]. Surgery is indicated when nonoperative treatment has failed. Noncompressive radiculopathy from diabetes, infectious (zoster, Lyme, etc.), granulomatous, and infiltrating neoplastic disorders has a worse prognosis.

TREATMENT: Surgical intervention considered with significant/severe [1] and progressive motor deficits and cauda equina syndrome [3] with bowel and bladder dysfunction. Symptoms limited to pain and sensory loss are managed medically [3]. Bed rest and anti-inflammatory agents (steroidal and/or nonsteroidal) with analgesics; muscle relaxants are helpful for significant spasms. Occasionally, oral steroids may reduce pain and inflammation from compression, but no controlled study exists to support this use; anecdotal reports suggest some usefulness. Slowly mobilize after 7–14 days. Generally, patients improve over 1–3 months with conservative treatment. If not, refer for surgical evaluation.

NCVS: This EMG/nerve conduction study shows an absent right peroneal motor response. The right tibial compound motor action potential (CMAP) amplitude is moderately reduced. The mild slowing right tibial

Clinical Electrophysiology. By © Peter W. Kaplan and Thien Nguyen. Published 2011 Blackwell Publishing Ltd.

Sensory nerve conduction

Nerve and site	Peak latency	Amplitude	Segment	Latency difference	Distance	Conduction velocity
Sural.R						
Point B	3.2 ms	14 µV	Lateral malleolus-Point B	2.2 ms	105 mm	48 m/s
Sural.L						
Point B	3.1 ms	11 µV	Lateral malleolus-Point B	2.2 ms	105 mm	48 m/s
Median.R						
Wrist	4.6 ms	11 µV	Digit II (index finger)-Wrist	3.5 ms	130 mm	49 m/s
Ulnar.R						
Wrist	3.1 ms	17 µV	Digit V (little finger)-Wrist	2.3 ms	110 mm	49 m/s

F-wave studies

Nerve	M-Letency	F-Letency
Tibial.R	6.8	66.4
Tibial.L	4.9	53.4
Peroneal.L	5.8	48.3
Median.L	3.2	25.4

Motor nerve conduction

Nerve and site	Latency	Amplitude	Segment	Latency difference	Distance	Conduction velocity
Peroneal.R						
Ankle	NR ms	mV	EDB-Ankle	ms	mm	m/s
Fibular Head	ms	mV	Ankle-Fibular Head	ms	mm	m/s
Pop Fossa	ms	mV	Fibular Head-Pop Fossa	ms	mm	m/s
Tibial.R						
ankle	4.7 ms	1.0 mV	AH-ankle	4.7 ms	mm	m/s
Tibial.L						
ankle	4.6 ms	16.9 mV	AH-ankle	4.6 ms	mm	m/s
Peroneal. L						
Ankle	5.3 ms	4.3 mV	EDB-Ankle	5.3 ms	mm	m/s
Fibular Head	12.8 ms	4.3 mV	Ankle-Fibular Head	7.5 ms	310 mm	41 m/s
Pop Fossa	14.2 ms	3.8 mV	Fibular Head-Pop Fossa	1.4 ms	100 mm	71 m/s
Median.L						
wrist	3.0 ms	4.4 mV	APB-wrist	3.0 ms	mm	m/s
antecubital	7.6 ms	3.4 mV	wrist-antecubital	4.6 ms	250 mm	54 m/s

Needle EMG examination

Muscle	Insertional Insertional	Spontaneous activity + Wave	Fibs	Fasc	Activation	Rate	Volitional MUAPs Duration	Amplitude	Config	Other
Gastrocnemius.R	Normal	+2	+2	None	MD	Rapid	SI	SI	Normal	
Tibialis anterior.R	Normal	+3	+3	None	GD	Rapid	SI	SI		
Rectus femoris.R	Normal	None	None	None						
Iliopsoas.R	Normal	None	None	None	GD	Rapid	Normal	Normal	Normal	Normal
Gluteus Maximus.R	Normal	+2	+2	None	MD	Rapid	SI	SI		
L5-paraspinous.R	Normal	+2	+2	None						
Gastrocnemius.L	Normal	None	None	None	MD	Rapid	SI	SI		

motor studies are appropriate for the significant loss in CMAP amplitude and probably related to loss of large, fast-conducting fibers. Together, these suggest several abnormalities: (1) L5 and S1 root lesion, (2) lumbosacral plexopathy, and (3) sciatic nerve lesion. Bilateral sural and superficial peroneal sensory studies are normal. Lesions of the sciatic nerve or the lumbosacral plexopathy are unlikely because they would cause reduced or absent superficial peroneal and sural sensory nerve action potential amplitudes. Needle EMG shows acute or chronic denervation/re-innervation in the L5–S1 myotome, and denervation in L5 paraspinous and gluteus medius and maximus muscles. These confirm an L5–S1 nerve root lesion by involvement of muscles outside sciatic nerve distribution and proximal to the lumbosacral plexus (i.e., paraspinous muscles). Hence, these findings indicate a severe right L5 radiculopathy with moderate involvement of the right S1 root.

REFERENCES:

1. Weinstein JN, Lurie JD, Tosteson TD, Skinner JS, Hanscom B, Tosteson AN, Herkowitz H, Fischgrund J, Cammisa FP, Albert T, Deyo RA. Surgical vs nonoperative treatment for lumbar disk herniation: The Spine Patient Outcomes Research Trial (SPORT) observational cohort. *JAMA* 2006;296:2451–2459.

2. Mazanec D, Okereke L. Interpreting the Spine Patient Outcomes Research Trial. Medical vs surgical treatment of lumbar disk herniation: Implications for future trials. *Cleve Clin J Med* 2007;74:577–583.

3. Nakagawa H, Kamimura M, Takahara K, Hashidate H, Kawaguchi A, Uchiyama S, Miyasaka T. Optimal duration of conservative treatment for lumbar disc herniation depending on the type of herniation. *J Clin Neurosci* 2007;14:104–109.

53. Guillain-Barré syndrome—demyelinating polyneuropathy

MICU, CICU, NICU

CLINICAL CORRELATES: Rapid onset of progressive (over days) ascending numbness, tingling of the extremities, weakness. Gait difficulty, shortness of breath, no bowel or bladder dysfunction. Recent flu-like illnesses.

ETIOLOGY: Demyelinating process.

CLINICAL EVALUATION: Normal cranial nerves. Extremity weakness—worse in the legs and worse proximally. Tendon reflexes absent. There may be mild distal pinprick and vibratory sensory loss; it is worse in the legs in comparison to the arms. Look for autonomic signs—variability in respiration, blood pressure, and cardiac rhythms.

ANCILLARY TESTING: Cervical spine MRI (myelopathy). Consider heavy metal screen, autoimmune panel, serum protein electrophoresis/immunofixation electrophoresis (SPEP/IFE), porphyria (delta-aminolevulinic acid (d-ALA), prophobilinogen (PBG)), serum CK level, pulmonary function test for indications of respiratory failure, and electrocardiogram (ECG) for cardiac assessment. Analysis of cerebrospinal fluid (CSF) for albuminocytologic dissociation—CSF protein raised typically 100–1000 mg/dL with normal or low CSF-WBC count.

DIFFERENTIAL DIAGNOSIS: Myelopathy, acute polyneuropathies, neuromuscular junction defect, or a myopathy. Acute spinal cord compression and acute transverse myelitis can resemble Guillain-Barré syndrome (GBS). The lack of a sensory level and sphincter dysfunction argues against a myelopathy. Normal cervical MRI excludes a myelopathy at this level. Neuromuscular junction problems including botulism, myasthenia gravis, and Lambert-Eaton myasthenic syndrome can cause acute weakness. Muscle disorders, for example, acute polymyositis and critical illness neuromyopathy, can result in diffuse paralytic weakness.

In this patient, there was rapid progression of acute diffuse weakness over a few days. Areflexia and mild sensory loss are out of proportion to the severity of weakness. Normal serum CK level, sensory loss, and electromyography (EMG) findings are not consistent with a myopathy or neuromuscular junction defect. Diminished sensory findings suggest an acute neuropathy.

Acute polyneuropathies include arsenic poisoning, n-hexane, or glue-sniffing neuropathy. Vasculitis, Lyme disease, tick paralysis, porphyria, sarcoidosis, leptomeningeal disease, paraneoplastic disease, and critical illness polyneuropathy cause peripheral neuropathy. Diffuse areflexia suggests demyelination. The diagnosis of GBS arises from a history of an acute monophasic illness with a rapidly progressive polyneuropathy, weakness, and areflexia. Weakness is usually proximal in the legs, but may begin in the face or arms (10%) [1]. Weakness varies from mild gait difficulty to complete paralysis including bulbar and respiratory muscle weakness. Thirty percent develop breathing difficulty, necessitating ventilatory support. Autonomic dysfunction occurs in 70%, with blood pressure instability, cardiac arrhythmias, ileus, and loss of sweating [2]. Severe dysautonomia must be monitored and may cause sudden death.

PROGNOSIS: Eighty percent recover completely or have minor deficits [3]; 15% persistent mild deficits (mild foot drop, balance problems, moderate weakness, painful dysesthesias); 3% remain wheelchair bound. Risk factors for poor prognosis: older age, rapid onset <7 days, ventilatory support, distal motor response amplitude reduction <20% normal; preceding diarrheal illness [4, 5]. About 2% of the patients develop chronic relapsing weakness of chronic demyelinating polyradiculopathy [6].

TREATMENT: ICU ventilatory and autonomic monitoring and support. American Academy of Neurology practice parameters recommend plasma exchange or intravenous immunoglobulins (IVIG) [7]. Plasmaphoresis and IVIG are

Clinical Electrophysiology. By © Peter W. Kaplan and Thien Nguyen. Published 2011 Blackwell Publishing Ltd.

Sensory NCS

Nerve/Sites	Rec. Site	Latency ms	Amplitude μV	Distance cm	Velocity m/s
L Median - Dig II					
1. Dig II	Wrist	2.05	17.0	12.5	61.0
L Ulnar					
1. Dig V	Wrist	2.20	6.8	11	50.0
L Sural					
1. Calf	Lat Mall	2.65	16.6	11	41.5

Motor NCS

Nerve/Sites	Rec. Site	Latency ms	Amplitude mV	Distance cm	Velocity m/s
L Median - APB					
1. Wrist	APB	4.15	9.4		
2. Elbow		8.45	4.9	26	60.5
3. Axilla		10.45	4.8	10	50.0
L Ulnar - ADM					
1. Wrist	ADM	3.10	4.6		
2. B.Elbow		6.60	2.9	21.5	61.4
3. A.Elbow		8.15	2.4	10	64.5
4. Axilla		10.45	0.8	9	39.1
L Peroneal - EDB					
1. Ankle	EDB	5.75	0.8		
2. FibHead		13.45	0.8	32.5	43.3
3. Knee		15.20	0.8	10	51.3
R Peroneal - EDB					
1. Ankle	EDB	5.80	2.5		

Needle EMG examination

Muscle	Insertional Insertional	Spontaneous Activity + Wave	Fibs	Fasc	Volitional MUAPs Activation	Rate	Duration	Amplitude	Config	Other
Iliopsoas.L	Normal	None	None	None	None	Normal	Normal	Normal	Normal	Normal
Rectus femoris.L	Normal	None	None	None	None	Normal	Normal	Normal	Normal	Normal
Tibialis anterior.L	Normal	None	None	None	None	Normal	Normal	Normal	Normal	Normal
Gastrocnemius (Medial head).L	Normal	None	None	None	None	Normal	Normal	Normal	Normal	Normal

F-Wave

Nerve	Fmin ms
L Peroneal	0.00
L Median	30.00

L Peroneal: No Response

R Peroneal: No Response

L Ulnar: No Response

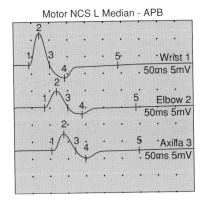

Motor NCS L Median - APB

of equivalent efficacy; combining the two treatments is not beneficial. Steroid treatment alone is not beneficial. During the recovery, patients often need intensive rehabilitation. Neuropathic pain may respond to antiseizure medications (gabapentin, pregabalin, topiramate, etc.), antidepressants (amitriptyline, duloxetine, etc.), or analgesics including opiate drugs.

NCV: This study shows prolonged bilateral peroneal distal latencies, absent left ulnar and bilateral peroneal F-wave latencies. Conduction blocks in the left ulnar nerve across the elbow and left median across the forearm. The asymmetrical nature of the abnormality suggests an acquired process. Concentric needle EMG is normal. The combined picture demonstrates a demyelinating polyneuropathy (e.g., early acute inflammatory demyelinating polyneuropathy or a GBS.

REFERENCES:

1. Ropper AH. The Guillain-Barré syndrome. *N Engl J Med* 1992;326:1130.

2. Zochodne DW. Autonomic involvement in Guillain-Barré syndrome: A review. *Muscle Nerve* 1994;17:1145.

3. Ropper AH, Wijdicks EFM, Truax BT. *Guillain-Barré Syndrome*. Philadelphia, PA: FA Davis 1991.

4. McKann GM, Griffin JW, Cornblath DR, Mellits ED, Fisher RS, Quashey SA. Plasmapheresis and Guillain-Barré syndrome: Analysis of prognostic factors and effect of plasmapheresis. *Ann Neurol* 1988;23:347.

5. Rees JH, Soudain SE, Gregson NA, Hughes RAC. Campylobacter jejuni infection and Guillain-Barré syndrome. *N Engl J Med* 1995;333:1374.

6. Asbury AK. New concepts of Guillain-Barré syndrome. *J Child Neurol* 2000;15:183.

7. Hughes RA, Wijdicks EF, Barohn R, Benson E, Cornblath DR, Hahn AF, Meythaler JM, Miller RG, Sladsky JT, Stevens JC; Quality Standards Subcommittee of the American Academy of Neurology. Practice parameter: immunotherapy for Guillain-Barré syndrome: Report of the Quality Standards Subcommittee of the American Academy of Neurology. *Neurology* 2003;61:736.

54. Myasthenia gravis—neuromuscular junction [1–4]

CICU, MICU, NICU

CLINICAL CORRELATES: Fatigable limb weakness, double vision, droopy eyelids, dysphagia, slurred speech, and facial weakness. Symptoms fluctuate.

ETIOLOGY: Neuromuscular junction defect such as Lambert-Eaton myasthenic syndrome, botulism, and myasthenia gravis (MG).

CLINICAL EVALUATION: Look for uni- or bilateral facial weakness, diplopia on sustained upward gaze, horizontal diplopia on sustained lateral gaze, ptosis on extended upward gaze, nasal speech, and weakness in the upper extremities, worse in the triceps muscle. Body and limb sensation and limb reflexes are normal.

ANCILLARY TESTING: Serum CK level, thyroid-stimulating-hormone (TSH), complete blood count, and metabolic panel. Brain MRI normal. Abnormal repetitive stimulation study—see below. Obtain respiratory function tests—negative inspiratory force (INF), first second of the forced exhalation (FEV1), vitalk capacity (VC)—anti-AChR and anti-MuSk antibodies. Consider chest CT with contrast to evaluate for thymoma.

DIFFERENTIAL DIAGNOSIS: Lambert-Eaton myasthenic syndrome, botulism, penicillamine-induced myasthenia, congenital myasthenic syndromes. Motor neuron disease is unlikely with normal reflexes, lack of fasciculation, young age.

MG usually affects the eye muscles early in the course with double vision and drooping of the lids, but can cause extremity weakness, difficulty speaking, swallowing, and breathing difficulty, necessitating ventilatory support. Weakness is often better after rest or in early morning; worse after exercise or later in the day. With MG, there is weakness and muscle fatigue (not "tiredness"). Electromyography (EMG)/NCV confirm postsynaptic neuromuscular disorder; sensitivity is about 75% [1].

PROGNOSIS: Nearly all are able to lead normal lives [3].

TREATMENT: Depending on presentation:

- Symptomatic treatment—Mestinon provides short-term benefit, lasting hours.
- Rapid immunomodulating treatment—Plasmapheresis and IVIg alter the abnormal antibody response.
- Chronic immunomodulating treatment—Corticosteroids and other immunosuppressive drugs suppress the abnormal antibody response, including the production of anti-AChR and anti-MuSK antibodies.
- Surgical removal of the thymus gland—The thymus gland is abnormal in about 75% of patients with MG. In about 15% there may be a thymus gland tumor, seen on CT or MRI of the chest. Surgical resection may provide benefit in patients without tumors [4].

NCVS: Sensory nerve action potentials and motor nerve conduction studies are normal. Repetitive nerve stimulation (RNS) at a rate of 3 Hz shows marked baseline decrements greater than 20% in three nerve–muscle pairs. An RNS study is considered positive if the decrement is greater than 10%. An improvement of the compound motor action potential decremental response (a smaller decrement of 13.6% compared with the decrement of 22.1% at rest) after brief exercise, reflecting postexercise facilitation. Concentric needle EMG is normal. These findings are consistent with a postsynaptic neuromuscular junction defect, such as MG.

REFERENCES:

1. Meriggioli MN, Sanders DB. Myasthenia gravis: Diagnosis. *Semin Neurol* 2004;24:31.
2. Vernino S, Lennon VA. Autoantibody profiles and neurological correlations of thymoma. *Clin Cancer Res* 2004;10:7270.
3. Drachman DB. Myasthenia gravis. *N Engl J Med* 1994; 330:1797.
4. Gronseth GS, Barohn RJ. Practice parameter: thymectomy for autoimmune myasthenia gravis (an evidence-based review): Report of the Quality Standards Subcommittee of the American Academy of Neurology. *Neurology* 2000;55:7.

Rep Nerve Stim

Muscle/Train	Amp mV	4-1 %	Lowest-1 %	Fac %	Area mVms	4-1 %	Lowerst-1 %	Fac %	Rate pps	Time
R Orb Oculi, CN VII										
Baseline	2.8	−22.1	−57.6	100	9.9	−29.1	−46.3	100	3	0:00:00
Post Exercise	3.3	−13.6	−60.7	117	9.7	−14.9	−37.3	98.2	3	0:00:44
@ 1:00	3.2	−24.3	−49	115	10.5	−29	−32.5	106	3	0:02:55
@ 2:00	3.4	−26.5	−71	122	10.8	−30.4	−70	109	3	0:03:59
@ 3:00	2.7	−25	−48.1	97.4	9.9	−33.7	−41.9	99.4	3	0:04:55
@ 5:00	3.0	−22	−44.9	110	10.1	−27.3	−30.3	102	3	0:07:56
L Orb Oculi, CN VII										
Baseline	3.9	−17.5	−36.9	100	10.3	−21.3	−21.3	100	3	0:00:00
R Trap, CN XI										
Baseline	12.0	−23.5	−27.4	100	75.6	−25.9	−32.3	100	3	0:00:00

EMG Summary Table		Spont			Recruit		Duration		Amplitude		PolyP	Other
		Fib	PSW	Fasc	MUs	FR	MUs	Dur	MUs	Amp	-	-
R. Deltoid, Axillary, C5-6		0	0	0	Nl	Nl	Nl	Nl	Nl	Nl	Nl	Nl

Rep Nerve Stim R Orb Oculi, CN VII

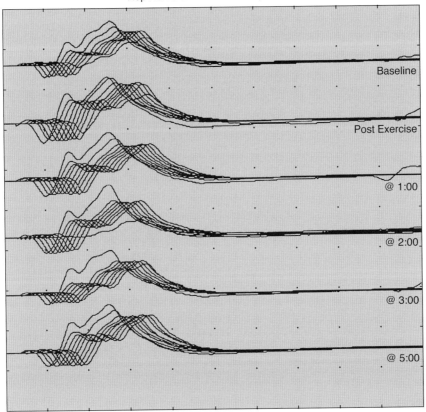

55. Myositis—irritable myopathy

CICU, MICU, NICU

CLINICAL CORRELATES: Slowly progressive limb weakness over weeks to months, swallowing difficulty, muscle pain, and respiratory symptoms. Purplish rash seen on the backs of the hands and across the face, and painful nodules.

ETIOLOGY: Myopathy.

CLINICAL EVALUATION: Look for slowly progressive proximal limb weakness, dysphagia, and respiratory weakness. Rash along the face, neck, chest, "shawl" distribution, arms, abdomen, thighs, patch on the thighs bilaterally. Normal sensation.

ANCILLARY TESTING: Complete blood count, creatine kinase (CK), lactate dehydrogenase, aldolase, and aspartate aminotransferase, erythrocyte sedimentation rate, anti-nuclear antibody, rheumatoid factor, anti-Ro, anti-La, anti-Sm, and anti-ribonucleoprotein antibodies. Myositis-specific autoantibodies directed against helicase (anti-Mi-2 antibodies), cytoplasmic RNA synthetases (anti-Jo-1 antibodies), other cytoplasmic proteins, ribonucleoproteins, and certain nuclear [1]. Muscle biopsy showing healthy muscle fibers surrounded and invaded by inflammatory cells ("primary inflammation"), worse perifascicularly in dermatomyositis. MRI of the limb to identify an optimal site for muscle biopsy. Malignancy screening is recommended due to its association with inflammatory myopathy, especially adult dermatomyositis. Evaluate respiratory function tests (i.e., INF, FEV1, and VC) for respiratory failure.

DIFFERENTIAL DIAGNOSIS: Muscle weakness with or without muscle enzyme elevation can be caused by myelopathy, lower motor neuron disease, radiculopathy,

plexopathy, neuropathy, myasthenia gravis, muscular dystrophies, and various metabolic, endocrine, inflammatory myopathy, and a variety of inherited, metabolic, drug-induced, endocrine, and infectious myopathies. Normal sensory modalities, reflexes, and an irritable myopathy on electromyogram (EMG) are against myelopathy, radiculopathy, plexopathy, and neuropathy. The absence of diurnal fluctuation, pupillary, ptosis, or ophthalmoplegic findings are against a neuromuscular junction disorder. Presentation of proximal muscle weakness and elevated muscle enzymes suggests a possible myopathy. Family history, sex (e.g., higher predominance in males), and distribution of weakness do not suggest a muscular dystrophy. The possibility of Churg–Strauss syndrome should be considered if there is eosinophilia. The distinctive purplish rash seen on the backs of the hands and across the face and painful nodules are most suggestive of dermatomyositis. Calcinosis, telangiectasias of scleroderma, and photosensitive rashes may be confused with systemic lupus erythematosus. A muscle biopsy can be helpful to make the definitive diagnosis.

PROGNOSIS: Long-term follow-up data on inflammatory myopathy are scant: 60% are chronic; 20% had polycyclic disease courses; and 20% had monophasic courses. Malignancy is seen with inflammatory myopathy, especially adult dermatomyositis. Myositis-specific autoantibody testing helps with prognosis and treatment [2, 3]: patients with anti-Jo-1 antibodies may have an incomplete response to treatment and a worse long-term weakness. Some with anti-signal recognition particle (SRP) antibodies have a fulminant onset of proximal muscle weakness, very high serum CK levels, and muscle biopsies that show muscle fiber necrosis and regeneration but little to no inflammation. Early glucocorticoid treatment may help some patients. With anti-Mi-2 antibodies (only seen in dermatomyositis (DM)), there may be a fulminant onset and florid cutaneous findings. They may respond well to treatment and have a good long-term prognosis

Clinical Electrophysiology. By © Peter W. Kaplan and Thien Nguyen. Published 2011 Blackwell Publishing Ltd.

Sensory nerve conduction

Nerve and site	Peak latency	Amplitude	Segment	Latency difference	Distance	Conduction velocity
Sural.R						
Point B	4.2 ms	11 µV	Lat malleolus-Point B	3.4 ms	120 mm	35 m/s
Sural.L						
Point B	3.7 ms	15 µV	Lat malleolus-Point B	2.8 ms	110 mm	39 m/s
Ulnar.L						
wrist	3.2 ms	14 µV	index finger-wrist	2.6 ms	140 mm	54 m/s
Median.L						
wrist	3.2 ms	14 µV	index finger-wrist	2.6 ms	140 mm	54 m/s

Motor nerve conduction

Nerve and site	Latency	Amplitude	Segment	Latency difference	Distance	Conduction velocity
Peroneal.R						
Ankle	5.4 ms	6.7 mV	EDB-Ankle	5.4 ms	mm	m/s
Fibular Head	13.2 ms	6.0 mV	Ankle-Fibular Head	7.8 ms	310 mm	40 m/s
Pop Fossa	15.2 ms	5.7 mV	Fibular Head-Pop Fossa	2.0 ms	90 mm	45 m/s
Tibial.R						
ankle	4.7 ms	15.7 mV	AH-ankle	4.7 ms	mm	m/s
Tibial.L						
ankle	4.6 ms	16.9 mV	AH-ankle	4.6 ms	mm	m/s
Peroneal.L						
Ankle	5.3 ms	4.5 mV	EDB-Ankle	5.3 ms	mm	m/s
Fibular Head	12.8 ms	4.3 mV	Ankle-Fibular Head	7.5 ms	310 mm	41 m/s
Pop Fossa	14.2 ms	3.8 mV	Fibular Head-Pop Fossa	1.4 ms	100 mm	71 m/s
Median.L						
wrist	3.0 ms	4.4 mV	APB-wrist	3.0 ms	mm	m/s
antecubital	7.6 ms	3.4 mV	wrist-antecubital	4.6 ms	250 mm	54 m/s
Ulnar.L						
wrist	3.0 ms	3.8 mV	wrist	3.0 ms	mm	m/s

Needle EMG data

		Insertional			Activation				
	Ins Act	Fibs	+Wave	Fasc	Amplitude	Duration	Config	Rate	Activation
Deltoid Middle	R Normal	1+	1+	None	SD	SD	Norm	None	EARLY
Biceps Brachii	R Normal	None	1+	None	MD	MD	Norm	None	EARLY
Triceps Med H	R Normal	None	1+	None	MD	MD	Norm	None	EARLY
Gastroc Med Hd	R Normal	None	None	None	Norm	Norm	Norm	None	Norm
Tibialis Ant	R Normal	None	None	None	MD	MD	Norm	None	Norm
Tibialis Ant	L Normal	None	None	None	Norm	Norm	Norm	None	Norm
Glut Med	L Normal	1+	1+	None	SD	SD	Norm	None	Norm

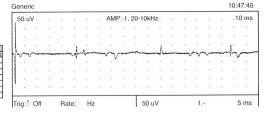

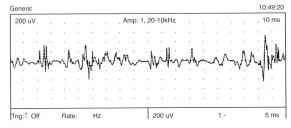

TREATMENT: Goals to improve muscle strength; avoid extramuscular complications. In DM, aim for resolution of cutaneous disease manifestations. There is no standard glucocorticoid regimen, but two general principles apply: (1) initiation of treatment with high doses for the first several months to establish disease control and (2) slow taper to the lowest effective dose for a total duration of therapy between 9 and 12 months.

Some clinicians initiate a glucocorticoid-sparing agent in a severely ill patient at the same time as steroid treatment is begun to reduce the cumulative dose of prednisone and diminish glucocorticoid-induced morbidity. Others reserve these agents for patients who fail treatment with glucocorticoids alone. The first-line glucocorticoid-sparing agent is usually either azathioprine or methotrexate. The response to azathioprine and methotrexate may take 4–6 months.

NCV: The sensory and motor nerve conduction studies are normal. Concentric needle EMG shows spontaneous activities (positive and fibrillation at rest), early recruitment, and many voluntary motor units with small amplitude and short duration consistent with a myopathic process such as an irritable myopathy. Consider dermatomyositis because of the rash. EMG can distinguish myopathic weakness from neuropathic disorders (e.g., motor neuron disease and myasthenia gravis) in which the EMG is normal. The EMG may be normal because of the patchy nature of muscle inflammation and placement of the needle electrode in an uninflamed site. The electromyographer should sample weak muscles and multiple muscles in several limbs before concluding there are no myopathic changes. The EMG usually shows irritability by (1) increased insertional activity and spontaneous fibrillations, (2) abnormal myopathic voluntary motor units—low amplitude, short-duration polyphasic motor potentials, and (3) high-frequency discharges consistent with early recruitment of motor units.

REFERENCES:

1. Targoff IN. Myositis specific autoantibodies. *Curr Rheumatol Rep* 2006;8:196.
2. Noss EH, Hausner-Sypeck DL, Weinblatt ME. Rituximab as therapy for refractory polymyositis and dermatomyositis. *J Rheumatol* 2006;33:1021.
3. Lambotte O, Kotb R, Maigne G, Blanc, FX, Goujard C, Delfraissy JF. Efficacy of rituximab in refractory PM. *J Rheumatol* 2005;32:1369.

56. Statin-induced myopathy—toxic myopathy/myalgia

ER, MICU

CLINICAL CORRELATES: Myalgia and muscle cramps, worse in the lower extremities. Taking statin drug for hyperlipidemia.

ETIOLOGY: Myopathy.

CLINICAL EVALUATION: Look for myalgias (with or without CK elevation), creatine kinase (CK) elevation, cramps, stiffness, muscle tenderness, exercise intolerance, proximal muscle weakness, often marked rhabdomyolysis with massive CK elevation, and occasionally life-threatening myoglobinuria with the risk of renal failure.

ANCILLARY TESTING: Complete blood count, CK, lactate dehydrogenase, aldolase, and aspartate aminotransferase, thyroid studies, erythrocyte sedimentation rate, anti-nuclear antibody, rheumatoid factor, anti-Ro, anti-La, anti-Sm, and anti-ribonucleoprotein antibodies. Myositis-specific autoantibodies directed against helicase (anti-Mi-2 antibodies), cytoplasmic RNA synthetases (anti-Jo-1 antibodies), other cytoplasmic proteins, ribonucleoproteins, and certain nuclear antigens [1]. Consider MRI of limbs to identify optimal site for muscle biopsy. Evaluate respiratory function tests (i.e., INF, FEV1, and VC) for respiratory failure.

DIFFERENTIAL DIAGNOSIS: Myopathy and myalgia symptoms can occur with inflammatory myopathies, lipid and glycogen storage disease, neuropathies and neuromuscular junction diseases, genetic dystrophies, toxic, metabolic, endocrine, and nutritional myopathies, polymyalgia rheumatica, and infection-associated myositis (viral, bacterial, and parasitic). The lack of long-track signs and fasciculations is against amyotrophic lateral sclerosis and other motor neuron diseases. The presence of the reflexes is against Guillain-Barré syndrome and similar neuropathies, including critical illness neuromyopathy. Disturbances of neuromuscular transmission often have pupillary, ptosis, or ophthalmoplegic findings. The lack of exposure to organophosphate, muscle spasm, or increased sweating would argue against organophosphate poisoning. The clinical presentation, elevated serum CK, and an irritable myopathy on electromyography (EMG) suggest a myopathy. With a history of exposure to simvastatin, statin-associated myopathy is the likely diagnosis [1, 2].

PROGNOSIS: Myalgias and weakness resolve; serum CKs normalize over days to weeks after stopping the drug. In 44 cases, 58% of patients had resolution of symptoms in less than 1 month and 93% had resolution in less than 6 months [2, 3].

TREATMENT: Failure to discontinue the statin or reduce the dose leads to progression of the myopathy and, in some patients, rhabdomyolysis. The myalgias may persist for months after drug discontinuation but eventually disappear in most patients. Clinical recovery with normalization of serum CK level follows drug discontinuation. No other treatment is necessary except for supportive care in patients with rhabdomyolysis.

Clinical Electrophysiology. By © Peter W. Kaplan and Thien Nguyen.
Published 2011 Blackwell Publishing Ltd.

Sensory nerve conduction

Nerve and site	Peak latency	Amplitude	Segment	Latency difference	Distance	Conduction velocity
Sural.R						
Point B	4.2 ms	14 µV	Lat malleolus-Point B	3.4 ms	120 ms	35 m/s
Sural.L						
Point B	3.7 ms	15 µV	Lat malleolus-Point B	2.8 ms	110 ms	39 m/s
Ulnar.L						
wrist	3.2 ms	14 µV	index finger-wrist	2.6 ms	140 ms	54 m/s
Median.L						
wrist	3.2 ms	13 µV	index finger-wrist	2.6 ms	140 ms	53 m/s

Motor nerve conduction

Nerve and site	Latency	Amplitude	Segment	Latency difference	Distance	Conduction velocity
Peroneal.R						
Ankle	5.4 ms	6.3 mV	EDB-Ankle	5.4 ms	mm	m/s
Fibular Head	13.2 ms	6.0 mV	Ankle-Fibular Head	7.8 ms	310 mm	40 m/s
Pop Fossa	15.2 ms	5.7 mV	Fibular Head-Pop Fossa	2.0 ms	90 mm	45 m/s
Tibial.R						
ankle	4.7 ms	16.0 mV	AH-ankle	4.7 ms	mm	m/s
Tibial.L						
ankle	4.3 ms	16.3 mV	AH-ankle	4.6 ms	mm	m/s
Peroneal.L						
Ankle	5.3 ms	4.5 mV	EDB-Ankle	5.3 ms	mm	m/s
Fibular Head	12.8 ms	4.3 mV	Ankle-Fibular Head	7.5 ms	310 mm	41 m/s
Pop Fossa	14.2 ms	3.8 mV	Fibular Head-Pop Fossa	1.4 ms	100 mm	71 m/s
Median.L						
wrist	3.0 ms	4.4 mV	APB-wrist	3.0 ms	mm	m/s
antecubital	7.6 ms	3.4 mV	wrist-antecubital	4.6 ms	250 mm	54 m/s
Ulnar.L						
wrist	3.0 ms	3.4 mV	wrist	3.0 ms	mm	m/s

Needle EMG data

		Insertional				Activation				
		Ins Act	Fibs	+Wave	Fasc	Amplitude	Duration	Config	Rate	Activation
Deltoid Middle	R	Normal	1+	1+	None	SD	SD	Norm	None	EARLY
Biceps Brachii	R	Normal	None	1+	None	MD	MD	Norm	None	EARLY
Triceps Med H	R	Normal	None	None	None	MD	MD	Norm	None	EARLY
Gastroc Med Hd	R	Normal	None	None	None	Norm	Norm	Norm	None	Norm
Tibialis Ant	R	Normal	None	None	None	MD	MD	Norm	None	Norm
Tibialis Ant	L	Normal	None	None	None	Norm	Norm	Norm	None	Norm
Glut Med	L	Normal	1+	1+	None	SD	SD	Norm	None	Norm
Iliopsoas	L	Normal	1+	1+	None	SD	SD	Norm	None	Norm

NCVs: Sensory and motor nerve conduction studies are normal. Needle EMG shows early recruitment and many voluntary motor units with short duration and low amplitude; some motor units are polyphasic. Low-grade spontaneous activities (i.e., fibrillation and positive waves) are noted in most muscles including the paraspinous muscles. These findings are consistent with a myopathy with mild irritability. Irritable myopathies include inflammatory myopathy, rapidly progressive muscle dystrophies, critical illness myopathy, parasitic myopathy (trichinosis), toxic myopathy, and myotubular myopathy. With a history of recent statin drugs, these findings suggest a statin-associated myopathy.

REFERENCES:

1. Thompson PD, Clarkson P, Karas RH. Statin-associated myopathy. *JAMA* 2003;289:1681.
2. Thompson PD, Clarkson PM, Rosenson RS. An assessment of statin safety by muscle experts. *Am J Cardiol* 2006;97:69C.
3. Hansen KE, Hildebrand JP, Ferguson EE, Stein JH. Outcomes in 45 patients with statin-associated myopathy. *Arch Intern Med* 2005;165:2671.

PART 5

The casebook of clinical/neurophysiology consults

57. Occipital blindness and seizures—why? [1–4]

CLINICAL CASE: A 43-year-old man with sickle cell disease and hypertension (203/110) was found to have a posterior reversible encephalopathy syndrome (PRES). He had a sudden onset of headache and total blindness while standing, followed by several convulsions. On MRI he had a posterior watershed T2-weighted serpiginous hypodensity and vasogenic edema.

CLINICAL EVALUATION: His eyes were open and he was unresponsive to voice and noxious stimuli, but with intact brainstem reflexes, and with a left gaze preference. Routine blood panel and cerebrospinal fluid were normal. The CT angiogram showed vasoconstriction of segments of the posterior cerebral artery territory.

TREATMENT: The patient received intensive treatment to lower his blood pressure using captopril and labetolol. He was given diazepam, followed by phenytoin. The PRES regressed.

DIAGNOSIS AND COMMENT: Visual cortex ischemia from hypertension-induced vasospasm with visual cortex seizures resulted in sudden blindness. PRES is an uncommon condition, more frequently seen in younger patients who sustain a sudden rise in blood pressure. It is seen in eclampsia, renal causes of hypertension, and after treatment with drugs used to suppress organ rejection, or for cancers (L-asparaginase, vincristine). Reversible occipital ischemia as may occur with eclampsia can result in reversible or irreversible occipital blindness. Vision can return because vasospasm abates with the lowering of the hypertension. Sickle cell disease can contribute to tissue ischemia because of the lower oxygen-carrying capacity of sickle cells and the anemia itself. Visual cortex seizures are a rare cause of reversible blindness.

The EEG shows a buildup of left occipital, high-frequency sharp waves evolving to slower rhythmic delta activity before stopping, indicating occipital seizures caused by PRES as the cause of his visual complaints

REFERENCES:

1. Bartynski WS. Posterior reversible encephalopathy syndrome, part I: Fundamental imaging and clinical features. *AJNR* 2008;29:1036–1042.
2. Williams J, Mozurkewich E, Chilimigras J, Van De Ven C. Critical care in obstetrics: Pregnancy-specific conditions. *Best Pract Res Clin Obstet Gynaecol* 2008;22(5):825–846.
3. Sawchuk KS, Chruchill S, Feldman E. Status epilepticus amauroticus. *Neurology* 1997;49:1467–1469.
4. Kaplan PW, Tusa RJ. Neurophysiologic and clinical correlations of epileptic nystagmus. *Neurology* 1993;43:2508–2514.

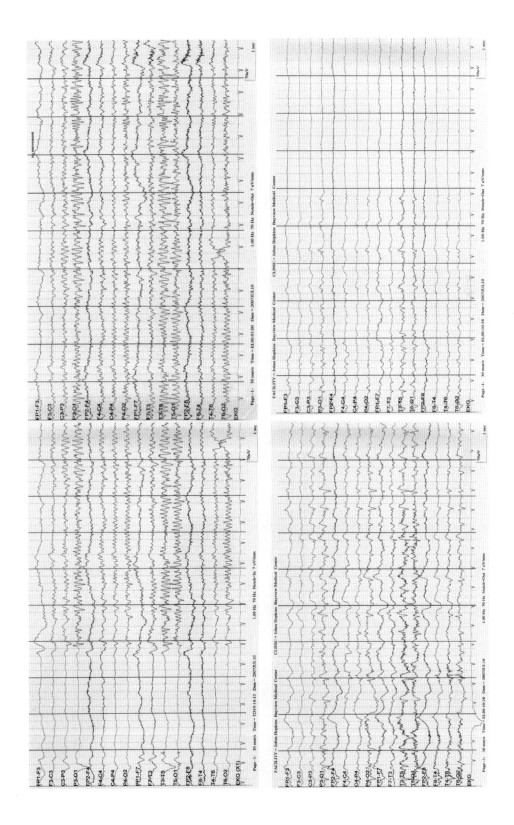

151

58. Unresponsiveness—coma, vegetative state, or locked-in state? [1–7]

CLINICAL CASE: This 34-year-old woman had headache and neck pain for 1 week, and then noted for 10 minutes that she could not move and felt tingling in her arms and legs. She called for an ambulance when she had difficulty breathing. In the ER, she was unresponsive to voice and stimulation, except to open or close her eyes, possibly to commands. Head CT scan showed no hemorrhage, and MRI/MRA and an angiogram showed a basilar artery occlusion with a stroke in the cerebellum and pons, and bilateral vertebral artery dissection. Intra-arterial TPA restored vertebrobasilar flow.

However, the next morning, her condition deteriorated; Doppler studies showed thrombosis of the proximal basilar artery and reversal of normal flow. MRI showed extension of a hemorrhagic infarction into the pons, cerebellar hemispheres, and midbrain with mild hydrocephalus.

From the EEG, is she in coma, a vegetative state (VS), or a locked-in state?

DEFINITIONS:

Coma—A clinical state of eyes-closed unresponsiveness from which the patient cannot be aroused (distinction from sleep) without purposeful response to external stimuli.

Vegetative state—The person is awake (eyes open) but unconscious.

Locked-in syndrome (LIS)—A de-efferented state: awake, conscious, but minimal evidence of reaction (vertical/horizontal eye movements to questions).

Clinical Electrophysiology. By © Peter W. Kaplan and Thien Nguyen. Published 2011 Blackwell Publishing Ltd.

TYPICAL FEATURES: The common theme is the paucity of reaction to stimuli. The patient may be in any of several states, ranging from conscious, clouded, minimally conscious to comatose along a continuum. Eyes may be open, closed, or open variably to command, stimuli, or open spontaneously. Movement below the neck is minimal or reflexive. See alternate sources for clinico/pathological information on these conditions.

CLINICAL EVALUATION: Examine brainstem reflexes, reactivity to stimuli (even minimal vertical eye movements to command). The assessment is largely directed at determining if there is a meaningful response to external stimuli that would suggest consciousness. Often more prolonged observation is needed, as families often report "meaningful" responses not seen by nurses and physicians. Assess Glasgow coma scale.

DIFFERENTIAL DIAGNOSIS: Minimally conscious state, VS, LIS, or coma.

DIAGNOSIS AND COMMENT: From the clinical description (the patient was unable to move, but was able to follow commands with eye movements as *yes/no* answers), and from an EEG confirming the presence of sleep and wake cycles, the diagnosis was LIS.

Patients with an obvious cause of unresponsiveness (CRA) still often pose diagnostic and prognostic challenges. In persistent vegetative state (PVS) or VS (<1 month) as well as with LIS, electrophysiology has yielded a wide range of findings, but few studies have been performed. Further, studies may show evolving results over time. A small series of eight patients had EEG patterns of alpha, slow activity, or triphasic waves across PVS and coma. fMRI has been found to differentiate conscious from unconscious patients, but clinical features still underpin the diagnosis of these various diagnostic entities.

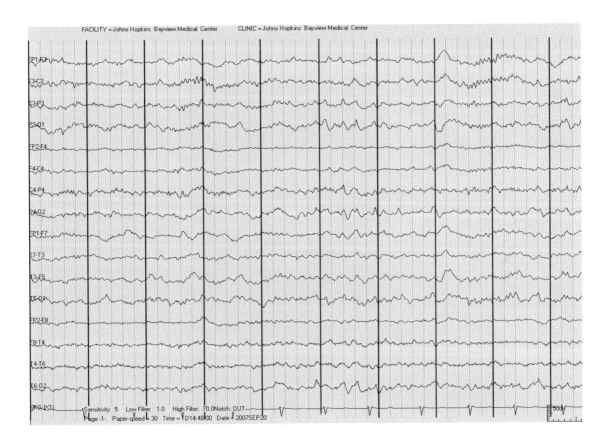

The EEG shows sleep spindles, diffuse theta, positive occipital sharp transients of sleep (POSTS) and vertex sharp waves. The pattern is reactive to stimuli producing alpha frequencies and abolition of sleep spindles and the POSTS.

REFERENCES:

1. Cartlidge N. States related to or confused with coma. *J Neurol Neurosurg Psychiatry* 2001;71(Supplement 1):i18–i19.
2. Gutling E, Isenmann S, Wichman W. Electrophysiology in the locked-in-syndrome. *Neurology* 1996;46:1092–1101.
3. Laureys S, Owen AM, Schiff ND. Brain function in coma, vegetative state, and related disorders. *Lancet Neurol* 2004;3:557–546.
4. Young GB. Major syndromes of impaired consciousness. In: Young GB, Ropper AH, Bolton CF (eds.), *Coma and Impaired Consciousness: A Clinical Perspective.* New York: McGraw-Hill 1998;39–78.
5. American Academy of Neurology Quality Standards Sub-committee. Practice parameters: Assessment and management of patients in the persistent vegetative state. *Neurology* 1995;45:1015–1018.
6. Bernat JL. Chronic disorders of consciousness. *Lancet* 2006;367:1181–1192.
7. Guérit JM. Neurophysiological patterns of vegetative and minimally conscious states. *Neuropsychol Rehabil* 2005;15:357–371.

59. Unresponsiveness—organic or psychogenic? [1, 2]

CLINICAL CASE: This 21-year-old patient was transported from an outside psychiatric institution with several weeks of history of florid hallucinations and a dream-like state, but no prior psychiatric history. After a week of headache, irritability, she had become delusional and unresponsive, becoming catatonic. At a psychiatric unit, she had a mild pneumonia; cerebrospinal fluid (CSF) showed 8 white blood cells (WBCs). We found her eyes opening to voice, intact brainstem reflexes, no vocalization, but posturing to pain. She had rigidity and catalepsy (waxy flexibility) of her arm, which remained transiently suspended in the air when placed there by the examiner. Initial EEG showed theta/delta activity, and treatment with valproate and lorazepam produced neither EEG nor clinical change. CSF repeat showed 13 WBCs, normal protein, and no bacterial growth. Tests for HSV, Epstein-Barr virus (EBV), cytomegalovirus, Varicella Zoster virus (VZV), enterovirus, fungi, *Bartonella*, *Brucella*, West Nile, Eastern, and Western equine encephalitis were normal. The brain MRI was normal.

DEFINITIONS:

Coma—A clinical state of eyes-closed unresponsiveness from which the patient cannot be aroused (distinction from sleep) without purposeful response to external stimuli.

Vegetative state—Awake (eyes open) but unconscious.
Locked-in syndrome (LIS)—De-efferented state: awake, conscious, but minimal evidence of reaction (vertical–horizontal eye movements to questions).
Catatonia—A state of psychic and motor unresponsiveness. It may be seen with schizophrenia, posttraumatic stress disorder, bipolar disease, depression, drug abuse,

and overdose. It can occur with strokes, metabolic and autoimmune conditions, encephalitis, adverse reactions to medications, and sudden withdrawal from benzodiazepines.

DIFFERENTIAL DIAGNOSIS: This includes encephalopathies. Coma, vegetative state (VS), minimally conscious state (MCS), LIS, and catatonia can be differentiated on the basis of clinical criteria by bedside testing. In coma, there is no evidence of clinical response to stimuli, including careful observation of eye movements to commands. LIS patients will have open eyes and can often make vertical eye movements to commands. A patient in MCS may require more prolonged observation, but again looking for evidence of some ability by the patient to follow commands, or answer (by signs or other). VS patients cycle through eyes-open wakefulness and sleep, but cannot react reproducibly to external commands. Catatonic patients from psychiatric causes may manifest eyes-closed resistance to opening or have occasional sideways glances. Patients with neuroleptic malignant (NMS) or serotonin syndrome (SS) are usually drowsier, are lethargic, will move purposefully to noxious stimuli, and have brainstem reflexes. Also, toxic, metabolic, and the NMS and SS can be confirmed by other clinical criteria, and tests for electrolyte, ammonia, liver function, and toxins.

ANCILLARY TESTING: Consider toxin screen, CPK, and liver enzymes. Imaging is rarely informative, except to exclude causes of coma, LIS, MCS, or VS. Obtain CSF for viral, fungal, bacterial, and paraneoplastic antigens.

DIAGNOSIS AND COMMENT: She had limbic status epilepticus from mycoplasma pneumonia. On admission, the patient was thought to have a diffuse encephalopathy/encephalitis given the nonlateralizing neurological examination, normal MRI of the brain, and the

Clinical Electrophysiology. By © Peter W. Kaplan and Thien Nguyen. Published 2011 Blackwell Publishing Ltd.

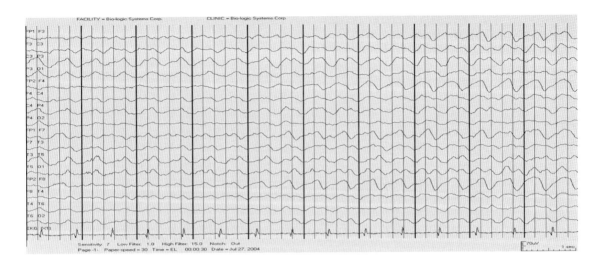

CSF studies showing less than 12 WBCs. All CSF, viral and autoimmune antigen panels were negative. Because of the pneumonia, she was tested for mycoplasmosis, which came back strongly positive. There are rare cases of nonconvulsive status epilepticus with mycoplasmosis, thought to arise from a cross-reactivity of brain structures with the mycoplasma surface antigens. This interaction may impair thalamocortical circuits. Of hospitalized patients with mycoplasma pneumonia, 7% can have central nervous system symptoms including seizures; overall 23% have serious sequelae. In this patient's case, she clinically and electroencephalographically had a limbic encephalopathy. The patient was treated with high-dose benzodiazepines, which normalized the rhythmic 2- to 4-Hz EEG pattern shown above. The patient returned to talking and following commands within 5 minutes. She was given a 4-week course of doxycycline for the mycoplasma pneumonia.

This EEG shows shifting rhythmic, monomorphic frontal, and diffuse theta/delta activity.

REFERENCES:

1. Koskiniemi M. CNS manifestations associated with *Mycoplasma pneumoniae* infections: Summary of cases at the University of Helsinki and review. *Clin Infect Dis* 1993;17:S52–S57.
2. Heatwole CR, Berg MJ, Henry JC, Hallman JL. Extreme spindles: A distinctive EEG pattern in *Mycoplasma pneumoniae* encephalitis. *Neurology* 2005;64:1096–1097.

60. Patient with a frontal brain tumor—psychiatric depression, paranoia, tumor growth, or status epilepticus? [1–4]

CLINICAL CASE: A 45-year-old man with a resected left frontal glioma had a history of complex partial seizures. An urgent consult was sought for the sudden onset of depressive thoughts, paranoia, and mild expressive aphasia with some waxing and waning of severity.

CLINICAL EVALUATION: He was alert but appeared puzzled, was searching for words, and frequently looked over at his wife. He would suddenly raise his eyebrows and was fidgety. MRI revealed no change from that of a few weeks before, prior to the behavioral change. The antiepileptic drug (AED) level was "subtherapeutic."

TREATMENT: His levetiracetam dosage was increased, and he was given 2 mg of lorazepam. The psychiatric, depressive, and inattention symptoms regressed.

DIAGNOSIS AND COMMENT: He had left frontal epileptiform activity causing hallucinations and paranoia, all of which regressed with AEDs.

Left frontal epileptic foci may produce bizarre psychiatric, complex motor, behavioral, and language disturbances. The depressive and paranoid features have long been recognized, but remain relatively rare phenomena.

Clinical Electrophysiology. By © Peter W. Kaplan and Thien Nguyen.
Published 2011 Blackwell Publishing Ltd.

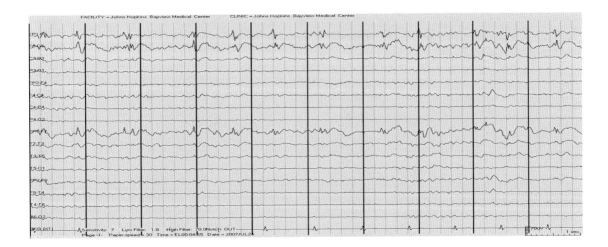

The EEG shows continuous left frontal epileptiform discharges at about 1 per second.

REFERENCES:

1. Thomas P, Zifkin B, Migneco O, Lebrun C, Darcourt J, Andermann F. Nonconvulsive status epilepticus of frontal origin. *Neurology* 1999;52:1174–1183.

2. Lim J, Yagnik P, Schraeder P, Wheeler S. Ictal catatonia as a manifestation of nonconvulsive status epilepticus. *J Neurol Neurosurg Psychiatry* 1986;49:833–836.

3. Rohr-Le Floch J, Gauthier G, Beaumanoir A. Confusional states of epileptic origin. Value of emergency EEG. *Rev Neurol* 1988;144:425–436.

4. Kaplan PW. Behavioral manifestations of non-convulsive status epilepticus. *Epilepsy Behav* 2002;3:122–139.

61. Patient with idiopathic generalized epilepsy on valproate—Metabolic encephalopathy or status epilepticus? [1–5]

CLINICAL CASE: A 68-year-old man with metastatic lung disease, and JME onset in his teens, had had several admissions in middle age for confusional states. During these events, he had been found to be in absence status (generalized nonconvulsive status epilepticus—GNSE) [1]. When he was on increased dosage of valproate because of seizures and status epilepticus that could not be controlled on other antiepileptic drugs, he had a waxing–waning confused state. EEG was performed and a basic metabolic panel was sent.

DIFFERENTIAL DIAGNOSIS: In this case, the differential considerations were among (a) toxic encephalopathy from medication, (b) compromised hepatic function with hyperammonemia, (c) an hypoxia from his compromised pulmonary status, or (d) GNSE for which he had been hospitalized many times before.

DIAGNOSIS AND COMMENT: He has a hyperammonemic encephalopathy from his valproate, and is not in nonconvulsive status (NCSE).

The EEG tracing now shows a slow background with triphasic waves (TWs) that are clearly distinguishable from his epileptiform discharges in the same tracing. Along with the raised ammonia, but unchanged liver enzymes, the diagnosis would be valproate-induced hyper-ammonemia (and not another cause of toxic/metabolic encephalopathy or NCSE).

TREATMENT: Valproate dosage was lowered as was his dietary protein, and his confusion and TWs regressed.

DISCUSSION: Epileptiform discharges are rarely seen along with TWs in the same patient. Much literature has been written on distinguishing characteristics between the two entities: TWs and spike-wave complexes (see the case with TWs). In the past there has been speculation that TWs were a reflection of epileptiform activity appearing in a severely compromised encephalopathic brain, hence the blunter, broader morphologies. There are however differences between them that include the reactivity of TWs to stimuli (increase TWs). Furthermore, TWs often appear in elderly patients with diffuse atrophy and white matter disease, as well as with a number of toxic/metabolic problems, suggesting a component of subcortical contribution to their appearance. As TWs do not appear in childhood, it is possibly because of the difference in thalamocortical transmission in the younger age group. Although still poorly understood, TWs may represent projected rhythms from the thalamus, which are altered along the path of the reverberating thalamo-cortical circuit.

Clinical Electrophysiology. By © Peter W. Kaplan and Thien Nguyen. Published 2011 Blackwell Publishing Ltd.

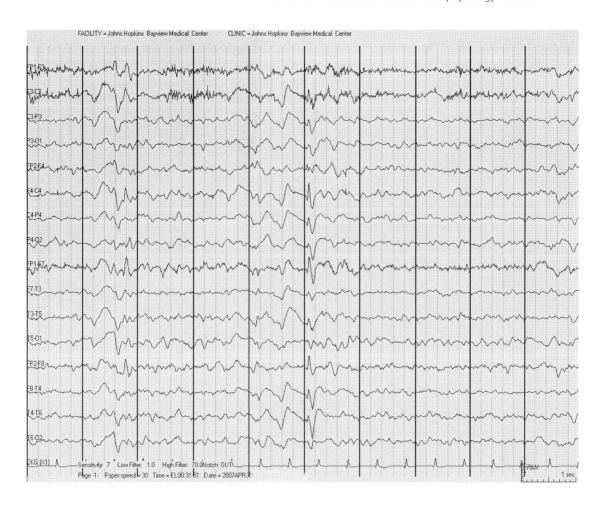

The EEG shows occasional generalized spike-slow wave discharges (see the end of the 2nd second and beginning of the 6th second of the EEG sample). These discharges were of short duration (spike to beginning of slow wave, with clear initial spike), and a field extending to the anterior frontal region, with occasional frontocentral phase reversals (similar to his interictal recordings). However, there are also now brief flurries of TWs on a slow background. The TWs are in the posterior centrofrontal region, have a minimal first phase, and a wider 1st to 2nd phase duration, with overall broader complexes than the epileptic discharge (see the 5th second). Hepatic aspartate aminotransferase and alanine aminotransferase (ALT) were unchanged from a baseline and from when he was previously fully alert, but the serum ammonia was 170 mg/mL.

REFERENCES:

1. Kaplan PW. Behavioral manifestations of non-convulsive status epilepticus. *Epilepsy Behav* 2002;3:122–139.
2. Baykan B, Gokyigit A, Gurses C, Eraksoy M. Recurrent absence status epilepticus: Clinical and EEG characteristics. *Seizure* 2002;11:310–319.
3. Thomas P, Valton L, Genton P. Absence and myoclonic status epilepticus precipitated by antiepileptic drugs in idiopathic generalized epilepsy. *Brain* 2006;129:1281–1292.
4. Sundaram MB, Blume WT. Triphasic waves: Clinical correlates and morphology. *Can J Neurol Sci* 1987;14:136–140.
5. Bahamon-Dussan JE, Celesia GG, Grigg-Damberger MM. Prognostic significance of EEG triphasic waves in patients with altered state of consciousness. *J Clin Neurophysiol* 1989;6:313–319.

62. Unresponsiveness—psychogenic, encephalopathy, or limbic encephalitis? [1–10]

CLINICAL CASE: A 51-year-old woman was transported from an outside hospital with a 10-month history of delirium, a dementia, partial seizures, sudden dystonic movements, and hyponatremia. Outside hospitals had diagnosed temporal lobe seizures on epilepsy monitoring, and had found normal thyroid antibodies, no 14-3-3 protein, normal paraneoplastic antibody panel, and a negative work-up for celiac disease, sarcoid, Whipple's disease, lupus, and systemic cancer. The MRI showed cortical laminar enhancement of the lateral, mesial, and insular temporal cortices more on one side than the other. Cerebrospinal fluid (CSF) protein was raised, cells normal, no viral antigens; serum sodium was 128. Examination revealed a minimental status examination of 26/30—marked and generalized memory impairment, but she could recite serial 7s and "WORLD" backward. She had bizarre, sudden grimacing with stiffening and asymmetric dystonic postures of both arms lasting less than 10 seconds of which she was unaware. She was on antiepileptic drugs and had tried a 3-day course of steroids.

DIFFERENTIAL DIAGNOSIS: Hashimoto's thyroid antibody encephalopathy, paraneoplastic encephalopathy, celiac disease, Whipple's disease, viral encephalitis, central nervous system lupus, nonconvulsive status, medication toxicity.

CLINICAL CORRELATION: There were no dystonic or other abnormal movements during the EEG.

DIAGNOSIS AND COMMENT: The patient had an antibody-mediated, voltage-gated anti-potassium channel nonparaneoplastic limbic encephalitis (VGKC) with seizures, paroxysmal dystonias, paranoia, confusion, and hyponatremia.

The constellation of partial seizures, movement disorder, and delirium in the absence of CSF cells or antibodies to viruses suggested a steroid-responsive thyroid antibody or paraneoplastic syndrome. This was tested for, but results were negative. Workups for other rare syndromes affecting cognition, causing encephalopathy, seizures, and movement disorders, such as Whipple's and celiac disease, were also negative. In addition, the presence of unexplained hyponatremia strongly suggested a potassium channel antibody-associated encephalopathy (VGKC)—an immunotherapy-responsive form of limbic encephalitis. High-dose steroids were started with a gradual taper; VGKC-Ab was remeasured; she was again screened for malignancy, and subsequently had IVIG and then plasmapheresis on subsequent relapses.

The hyponatremia from syndrome of inappropriate antidiuretic hormone (SIADH) is well recognized in this condition and improves with immunotherapy-induced fall in VGKC-Ab.

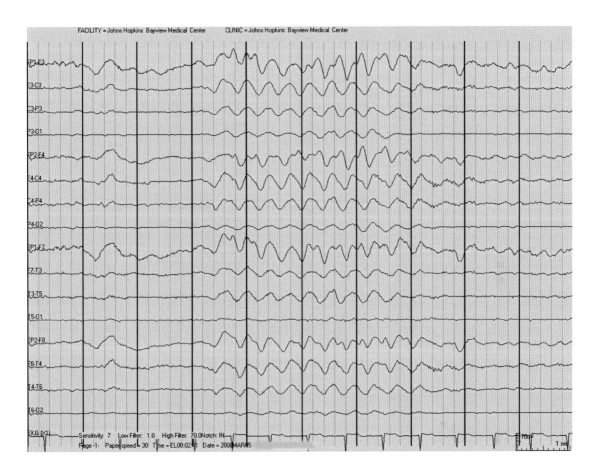

FACILITY = Johns Hopkins Bayview Medical Center   CLINIC = Johns Hopkins Bayview Medical Center

This EEG shows runs of frontal 2–3 Hz rhythmic, occasionally notched delta activity, not clearly related to sleep, arousal, or change in clinical state. There is a low-voltage fast background EEG pattern.

REFERENCES:

1. Vincent A, Buckley C, Schott J, Baker I, Dewar BK, Detert N, Clover L, Parkinson A, Bien CG, Omer S, Lang B, Rossor MN, Palace J. Potassium channel antibody-associated encephalopathy: A potentially immunotherapy-responsive form of limbic encephalitis. *Brain* 2004;127:701–712.
2. Alamowitch S, Graus F, Uchuya M, Ren R, Bescansa E, Delattre JY. Limbic encephalitis and small cell lung cancer. Clinical and immunological features. *Brain* 1997;120:923–928.
3. Brierley JB, Corsellis JAN, Hierons R, Nevin S. Subacute encephalitis of later adult life mainly affecting the limbic areas. *Brain* 1960;83:357–368.
4. Chong JY, Rowland LP, Utiger RD. Hashimoto encephalopathy: Syndrome or myth? *Arch Neurol* 2003;60:164–171.
5. Dunstan EJ, Winer JB. Autoimmune limbic encephalitis causing fits, rapidly progressive confusion and hyponatremia. *Age Aging* 2006;35:536–537.
6. Bataller L, Kleopa KA, Wu GF, Rossi JE, Rosenfeld MR, Dalmau J. Autoimmune limbic encephalitis in 39 patients: Immunophenotypes and outcomes. *J Neurol Neurosurg Psychiatry* 2007;78:381–385.
7. Stubgen JP. Nervous system lupus mimics limbic encephalitis. *Lupus* 1998;7:557–560.
8. Iizuka T, Sakai F, Ide T, Monzen T, Yoshii S, Iigaya M, Suzuki K, Lynch DR, Suzuki N, Hata T, Dalmau J. Anti-NMDA receptor encephalitis in Japan. *Neurology* 2008;70:504–511.
9. McKeon A, Marnane M, O'Connell M, Stack JP, Kelly PJ, Lynch T. Potassium channel antibody-associated encephalopathy presenting with a frontotemporal dementia-like syndrome. *Arch Neurol* 2007;64:1528–1530.
10. Thieben MJ, Lennon VA, Boeve BF, Aksamit AJ, Keegan M, Vernino S. Potentially reversible autoimmune limbic encephalitis with neuronal potassium channel antibody. *Neurology* 2004;62:1177–1182.

63. Respiratory weakness—toxic or metabolic?

CLINICAL CASE: A 26-year-old woman was admitted to the hospital with nausea, vomiting, abdominal pain, and weight loss for 3 weeks. She developed lower extremity weakness with paresthesias in her feet 2 days prior to admission. On the day of admission, she was unable to move her legs and had worsening weakness in the upper extremities. She could not feel her lower extremities. One day into her hospitalization, she became increasingly confused. She later developed respiratory failure. There was no bowel or urinary incontinence. At the time of her hospital admission, examination showed 0/5 strength in the legs, 4/5 in the proximal upper extremities, and 4−/5 distally. Reflexes were diffusely depressed. There was markedly reduced pinprick sensation in the legs and loss of vibratory and proprioception sensation; no Babinski's sign. Cervical and thoracic MRIs were normal, as were CPK, complete blood count, and complete metabolic panel. Heavy metal screen and cerebrospinal fluid were normal.

DIFFERENTIAL DIAGNOSIS: The differential diagnosis includes not only acute polyneuropathies, but also myelopathy, neuromuscular junction defect, and myopathy. Acute polyneuropathies include arsenic poisoning, n-hexane or glue-sniffing neuropathy, vasculitis, Lyme disease, tick paralysis, porphyria, sarcoidosis, leptomeningeal disease, paraneoplastic disease, and critical illness polyneuropathy. Arsenic poisoning, porphyria, and acute severe vasculitic neuropathy should be considered. An axonal polyneuropathy is not consistent with classic Guillain-Barré syndrome (GBS), but an axonal form acute motor axonal neuropathy (AMAN) still needs to be considered. The abdominal pain and psychosis suggest possible acute intermittent porphyria (AIP). Absent Babinski's signs, lack of a sensory level, and no bowel/urinary

incontinence are against a myelopathy. The spine MRI is also normal. The sensory finding is against a motor neuron disease. Neuromuscular junction disorders may present acutely, but usually cause bulbar weakness, papillary dysfunction, ptosis, or ophthalmoplegia. The sensory loss and hyporeflexia also argue against myasthenia gravis. There is no exposure to suggest organophosphate poisoning. Myopathies are also unlikely because of the hyporeflexia and sensory loss. In summary, this patient has a rapidly progressing axonal polyneuropathy such as arsenic poisoning, porphyria, GBS (i.e., AMAN), or acute severe vasculitic neuropathy. The abdominal pain and psychosis possibly suggest porphyria.

DIAGNOSIS AND COMMENT: The asymmetric, axonal motor polyneuropathy with abdominal pain, psychosis and raised d-ALA and porphobilinogen indicate AIP. Patients with AIP usually present with abdominal pain, psychiatric symptoms such as hysteria, and mainly axonal motor polyneuropathies. Most patients are completely free of symptoms between attacks. AIP displays neurovisceral symptoms but no skin manifestations. There may be autonomic neuropathies (e.g., constipation, colicky abdominal pain, vomiting, and hypertension), peripheral neuropathy, seizures, delirium, coma, and depression. The abdominal pain is severe and lasts for several days. Severe abdomen pain of short (<1 day) duration or chronic abdominal pain is unusual. The pain is often epigastric and colicky in nature. Constipation is common and can be very severe. Frequently, nausea and vomiting are present. AIP patients may have central nervous system signs, consisting of seizures, mental status changes, cortical blindness, coma, and psychiatric symptoms. Finally, patients often experience peripheral neuropathies that are predominantly motor and can mimic GBS. The weakness usually starts in the lower limbs and ascends, but neuropathies can be observed in any nerve distribution. Areflexia or hyporeflexia is often present on examination. Patients also may have cortical blindness. Diffuse pain,

Clinical Electrophysiology. By © Peter W. Kaplan and Thien Nguyen. Published 2011 Blackwell Publishing Ltd.

Needle EMG Data:

		Insertional				Activation				
		Ins Act	Fibs	+Wave	Fasc	Amplitude	Duration	Config	Rate	Activation
Deltoid Middle	R	Increased	1+	1+	None	SI	SI	Norm	None	Reduced
Biceps Brachii	R	Increased	None	1+	None	Norm	Norm	Norm	None	Reduced
Triceps Med H	R	Normal	None	None	None	Norm	Norm	Norm	None	Norm
Gastroc Med Hd	R	Normal	None	None	None	Norm	Norm	Norm	None	Norm
Tibialis Ant	R	Increased	None	1+	None	Norm	Norm	Norm	None	Norm
Tibialis Ant	L	Increased	None	1+	None	Norm	Norm	Norm	None	Norm
Glut Med	L	Increased	1+	1+	None	SI	SI	Norm	None	Reduced

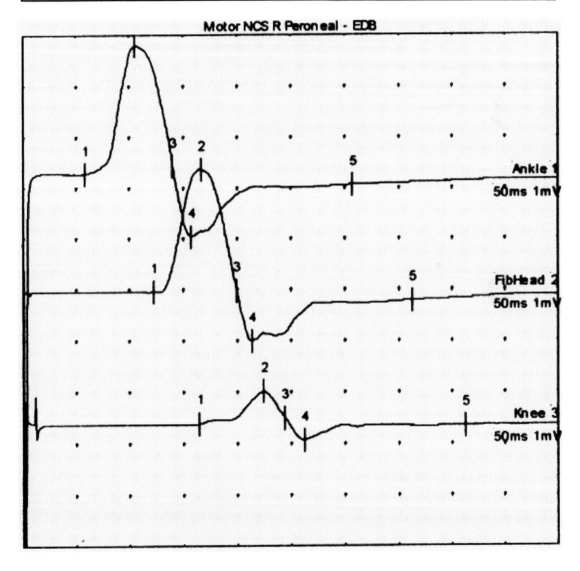

especially in the upper body, can be observed. Patients may develop autonomic neuropathies, such as hypertension and tachycardia. The fundamental step in diagnosing AIP is to demonstrate increased urinary porphobilinogen secretion, particularly during an attack. Between attacks, the enzyme uroporphyrin-1-synthetase may be decreased.

PROGNOSIS: Most patients (60–80%) have a single acute attack. Avoidance of precipitating factors helps prevent attacks [1, 2].

TREATMENT: The treatment for acute attacks of porphyria is to decrease heme synthesis and reduce the production of porphyrin precursors [3]. High doses of glucose (400 g/day) can inhibit heme synthesis and are useful for treatment of mild attacks. Severe attacks, especially those with severe neurologic symptoms, should be treated with hematin in a dose of 4 mg/kg per day for 4 days. Pain control is best achieved with narcotics. Laxatives and stool softeners should be administered with the narcotics to avoid exacerbating a coexisting constipation. The patient should receive a high-carbohydrate diet during the attack. If the patient is unable to eat, intravenous glucose should be administered. Between attacks, eating a balanced diet is more important than eating one rich in glucose.

NCVs: Bilateral sural sensory nerve action potential amplitudes were mildly reduced. There was conduction block in the left peroneal nerve across the knee, found again 1 week later, with an absent left peroneal response. Left ulnar, median, and radial sensory responses were normal; both peroneal and tibial compound motor action potential (CMAP) amplitudes were reduced along with left ulnar and median CMAP amplitudes. Right ulnar and median motor studies were normal. Needle electromyography showed acute denervation in the lower and upper extremities. These findings are indicative of an asymmetric, motor polyneuropathy with predominantly axonal features

REFERENCES:

1. Anderson KE, Bloomer JR, Bonkovsky HL, Kushner JP, Pierach CA, Pimstone NR, Desnick RJ. Recommendations for the diagnosis and treatment of the acute porphyrias. *Ann Intern Med* 2005;142(6):439–450.
2. Kauppinen R, Mustajoki P. Prognosis of acute porphyria: Occurrence of acute attacks, precipitating factors, and associated diseases. *Medicine (Baltimore)* 1992;71(1): 1–13.
3. Mustajoki P, Tenhunen R, Pierach C, Volin L. Heme in the treatment of porphyrias and hematological disorders. *Semin Hematol* 1989;26:1.

Sensory Nerve Conduction:

Nerve and Site	Peak Latency	Amplitude	Segment	Latency Difference	Distance	Conduction Velocity
Sural.R						
Point B	3.2 ms	8 μV	Lateral malleolus-Point B	2.2 ms	105 mm	48 m/s
Sural.R						
Point B	3.1 ms	7 μV	Lateral malleolus-Point B	2.1 ms	105 mm	48 m/s
Median.R						
Wrist	4.1 ms	17 μV	Digit II (index finger)-Wrist	2.5 ms	130 mm	52 m/s
Ulnar.R						
Wrist	3.1 ms	11 μV	Digit V (little finger)-Wrist	2.1 ms	110 mm	50 m/s
Radial.R						
Forearm	1.7 ms	30 μV	Dorsum of hand-Forearm	1.7 ms	100 mm	59 m/s

Motor Nerve Conduction:

Nerve and Site	Latency	Amplitude	Distance	Conduction Velocity
Peroneal.R				
Ankle	5.4 ms	1.2 mV	mm	m/s
Fibula (head)	10.7 ms	1.0 mV	240 mm	45 m/s
Popliteal fossa	12.5 ms	0.6 mV	90 mm	50 m/s
Tibial.R				
Ankle	6.1 ms	1.0 mV	mm	m/s
Tibial. L				
Ankle	5.4 ms	1.2 mV	mm	m/s
Peroneal.L				
Fibula (head)	3.0 ms	1.6 mV	mm	m/s
Popliteal fossa	4.6 ms	2.1 mV	90 mm	56 m/s
Median.R				
Wrist	3.3 ms	6.2 mV	mm	m/s
Antecubital	7.7 ms	5.1 mV	270 mm	61 m/s
Ulnar.R				
Wrist	3.4 ms	8.4 mV	mm	m/s
Below elbow	7.7 ms	7.1 mV	210 mm	51 m/s
Above elbow	9.1 ms	8.4 mV	70 mm	50 m/s
Median.L				
Wrist	4.1 ms	2.5 mV	mm	m/s
Antecubital	8.9 ms	2.3 mV	260 mm	54 m/s
Ulnar.L				
Wrist	2.7 ms	2.4 mV	mm	m/s
Below elbow	6.6 ms	2.1 mV	200 mm	52 m/s
Above elbow	8.1 ms	2.0 mV	70 mm	50 m/s

64. Failure to wean from a ventilator/internal ophthalmoplegia—bulbar dysfunction, neuromuscular junction problem, or polyneuropathy?

CLINICALCASE: A 35-year-old man woke up with double vision, and by the evening, had droopy eyelids and blurred vision. The next morning, he had nausea and vomiting followed by slurred speech and swallowing difficulty. Examination showed bilateral external ophthalmoplegia and ptosis. Pupils were dilated and unreactive to light or attempted accommodation. Corneal reflexes were depressed. There was bilateral facial weakness of the upper and lower face; tongue was weak without fasciculation. There was no gag. Neck flexion and extension (Medical Research Council 4/5) and pelvic and shoulder girdle muscle (5−/5) were mildly weak. Tendon reflexes were depressed (1/4). Body and limb sensation, and limb reflexes were normal. The creatine kinase (CK), complete blood count, and metabolic panel were normal; brain MRI was normal.

DIFFERENTIAL DIAGNOSIS: Viral syndrome, encephalitis, Guillain-Barré syndrome, and acute neuropathies are the most common. Myasthenia gravis, botulism, inflammatory myopathy, diabetic complications, hyperemesis gravidarum with hypokalemia, hypothyroidism, and laryngeal trauma are rarer considerations.

The progression of symptoms over several days suggests a subacute process, but the presence of reflexes and normal sensory examination are against Guillain-Barré syndrome and acute neuropathies. The prominent involvement of bulbar weakness, normal serum CK elevation, and electromyography (EMG) findings are not seen with a myopathy. A neuromuscular junction dysfunction remains high on the differential diagnosis. The lack of fatigable weakness, depressed corneal reflexes, and unreactive pupils support a diagnosis of a presynaptic neuromuscular junction dysfunction, namely botulism in this case. This is in agreement with the modest increment on repetitive stimulation at high frequency and after a short period of exercise.

DIAGNOSIS AND COMMENT: The compound muscle action potential (CMAP) increment with rapid, repetitive stimulation is modest (30–100%) in botulism in comparison to marked increment (usually >200%) in Lambert-Eaton myasthenic syndrome. The above findings are consistent with botulism.

Botulism is rare but potentially fatal. Botulism should be suspected with (1) rapid, descending muscular weakness (ocular to bulbar to extremities), (2) subacute bilateral ophthalmoplegia, particularly with pupil dilatation, (3) generalized weakness associated with autonomic symptoms, and (4) a history of contaminated food ingestion or a wound.

PROGNOSIS: Before 1950, mortality with botulism was reported to be about 60% [1]. It is now less than 8% in the USA because of critical care and respiratory support [2,3]. Heightened awareness, better recognition, and earlier administration of antitoxin also play a role in this improvement. Recovery is usually protracted, and may continue for as long as 5 years.

TREATMENT: Supportive treatment is essential. This includes artificial ventilation, feeding, prophylaxis for deep vein thrombosis, and physical therapy for prevention of muscle and tendon contractures. Efforts to neutralize the toxin should be immediate with trivalent antitoxin (A, B, and E)—most effective early in the disease—unlikely to be effective more than 3 days after exposure [4]. Cleansing the gastrointestinal tract by enema or lactulose and neomycin are useful, especially in infants. Guanidine and 3,4-diaminopyridine can help.

Clinical Electrophysiology. By © Peter W. Kaplan and Thien Nguyen.
Published 2011 Blackwell Publishing Ltd.

Sensory nerve conduction

Nerve and site	Peak latency	Amplitude	Segment	Latency difference	Distance	Conduction velocity
Sural.R						
Point B	3.2 ms	14 µV	Lateral mallcolus-Point B	2.2 ms	105 mm	48 m/s
Median.R						
Wrist	4.1 ms	11 µV	Digit II (index finger)-Wrist	2.5 ms	130 mm	52 m/s
Ulnar.R						
Wrist	3.1 ms	17 µV	Digit V (little finger)-Wrist	2.1 ms	110 mm	50 m/s

Rep nerve stim

Muscle / train	Amp mV	4-1 %	Lowest-1 %	Fac %	Area mVms	4-1 %	Lowerst-1 %	Fac %	Rate pps	Time
L ADM, Uln, C8-T1										
Baseline	1.1	15.8	−3.6	100	3.0	111	−32.3	100	50	0:00:00
L ADM, Uln, C8-T1										
Baseline	0.6	44.7	−0.3	100	1.6	99.6	−27.6	100	50	0:00:00
L ADM, Uln, C8-T1										
Baseline	0.5	18.4	67.3	100	0.8	2.1	−28.1	100	50	0:00:00
L APB, Med, C8-T1										
Baseline	0.7	2.1	−0.2	100	2.2	5.5	−17.4	100	50	0:00:00

EMG summary table	Spent			Recruit		Duration		Amplitude		PolyP	Other
	Fib	PSW	Fasc	MUs	FR	MUs	Dur	MUs	Amp	–	–
L. Deltoid, Axillary, C5-6	0	0	0	Early	NI	Most	2−	Most	2−	Most	NI
L. Biceps, Musculoe, C5-6	NR	NR	NR	Early	–	Most	3−	Most	3−	Most	NI

Motor NCS (Demy)

Nerve / sites	Lat ms	Amp mV	Rel Amp %	Dist cm	Vel m/s	Area mVms	Rel Area %	Dur ms	Rel Dur %
L Median - APB									
Wrist	2.70	0.8	100			1.9	100	4.35	100
Elbow	4.25	0.4	49.6	7	45.2	1.1	59.8	5.00	115
L Ulnar - ADM									
Wrist	2.70	0.7	100			1.1	100	5.00	100
B.Elbow	6.35	0.9	134	9	24.7	1.7	155	4.05	81
L Peroneal - EDB									
Ankle	2.55	0.7	100			1.3	100	2.80	100

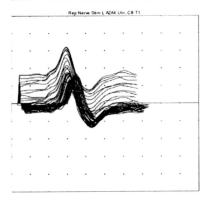

Rep Nerve Stim L ADM, Uln, C8-T1

NCVs: Sensory nerve action potentials are normal. CMAP amplitudes are mildly reduced. Repetitive stimulation at 3 Hz of the median and facial nerve at rest shows a 13% decrement. There is an 80% increment of the median CMAP amplitude after rapid, repetitive stimulation (50 Hz). Similarly, there is a 70% increment of the median CMAP recording at the abductor pollicis brevis muscle after a short period of exercise. Needle EMG of the selected muscles is normal. These findings are consistent with a neuromuscular junction disorder of the presynaptic type, supported by postexercise CMAP facilitation and a significant increment (>50%) of the CMAP amplitude after rapid, repetitive stimulation of the motor nerves.

REFERENCES:

1. Centers for Disease Control and Prevention. *Botulism in the United States 1899–1996*. Handbook for Epidemiologists, Clinicians and Laboratory Workers.

2. Abrutyn E. Botulism. In: Fauci AS, Isselbacher KJ, Braunwald E (eds.), *Principles of Internal Medicine*, 14th edn. New York: McGraw-Hill 1998;904.

3. Varma JK, Katsitadze G, Moiscrafishvili M, Zardiashvili T, Chokheli M, Tarkhashvili N, Jhorjholiani E, Chubinidze M, Kukhalashvili T, Khmaladze I, Chakvetadze N, Imnadze P. Hoekstra M, Sobel J, Hennessy TW, Rotz LD. Signs and symptoms predictive of death in patients with foodborne botulism–Republic of Georgia, 1980–2002. *Clin Infect Dis* 2004;39:357.

4. Arnon SS, Schechter R, Maslanka SE, Jewell NP, Hatheway CL. Human botulism immune globulin for the treatment of infant botulism. *N Engl J Med* 2006;354(5):462–471.

65. Progressive sensory loss and painful gait—radiculopathy, toxic, infectious neuropathy, or myopathy?

CLINICAL CASE: A 27-year-old man with HIV has several weeks of progressive leg pain and is now unable to walk. Examination shows that he has painful feet (including soles), sensitive to light touch, with a symmetric distal sensory loss to all modalities just below the knee. There is mild distal weakness of ankle dorsiflexion and plantar flexion. Deep tendon reflexes are absent in the ankles and reduced in the knees. There is normal CPK, complete blood count and metabolic process; cerebrospinal fluid shows a mild pleocytosis and protein elevation.

DIFFERENTIAL DIAGNOSIS: The differential for painful neuropathy includes acute inflammatory demyelinating polyradiculoneuropathy, diabetic neuropathy, HIV-1-associated multiple mononeuropathies, nutritional neuropathy, toxic neuropathy, other HIV-related neuropathies (differentiated by HIV-associated distal painful sensory, neuropathy's slower progression), alcoholic neuropathy, and a metabolic neuropathy. A paraneoplastic sensory neuropathy, paraproteinemic neuropathy, cytomegalovirus-related mononeuropathy, human T-cell leukemia virus type 2 (HTLV-2)-related neuropathy, and vasculitic neuropathy are less common.

DIAGNOSIS AND COMMENT: HIV-positive serology, neuropathic pain, and paresthesias with gradual spreading proximally in the lower extremities should suggest HIV-associated distal symmetric peripheral neuropathy (DSPN).

There are a number of distinctive neuropathic syndromes, which can be classified according to the timing of their appearance during HIV infection, their etiology, and whether they are primarily axonal or demyelinating. The most common of these is peripheral neuropathy, also referred to as DSPN. DSPN usually manifests as bilateral tingling and numbness in the toes. The neuropathy gradually spreads proximally in the lower extremities,

with only rare involvement of the upper extremities. The spread of sensory symptoms usually occurs over weeks to months. Neuropathic pain is common and may be the presenting symptom. Neurologic examination shows sensory loss to all sensory modalities (vibration, pinprick, temperature) in a stocking distribution, while deep tendon reflexes are reduced or absent at the ankles and occasionally at the knees in more severe cases. Distal weakness in the lower extremities can occur, although most patients have only sensory symptoms and signs. Sensory findings in the hands are more commonly associated with drug toxicity. HIV-related DSPN may evolve from painful to painless numbness. Skin biopsy for epidermal nerve fiber density analysis has been shown to correlate with neuropathy severity, level of neuropathic pain, and sensory amplitudes on electrodiagnostic studies. Nerve biopsy is not usually required but is occasionally performed in severe cases to exclude a concurrent mononeuropathy multiplex. Biopsies show axonal loss with frequent foci of inflammation in the endoneurium or around perineurial blood. Other HIV-associated neuropathies include acquired inflammatory demyelinating polyradiculoneuropathy, cauda equina syndrome, diffuse infiltrative lymphocytosis syndrome, autonomic neuropathy, mononeuropathies, herpes zoster radiculitis, and sensory ganglionopathy.

PROGNOSIS: HIV-associated distal painful neuropathy is a progressive disease. The effect of highly active antiretroviral therapy (HAART) on the distal symmetrical polyneuropathy is unclear, although there is some evidence showing improved quantitative sensory measures in patients responding to HAART [1, 2].

TREATMENT: Treatment is directed at the cause and the symptoms. Treatment of the cause includes discontinuing potentially neurotoxic drugs (i.e., stavudine (d4T) or didanosine (ddI) or thalidomide). Management of DSPN is symptomatic, aimed at the painful dysesthesias. Gabapentin, topiramate, antidepressants topical

Clinical Electrophysiology. By © Peter W. Kaplan and Thien Nguyen. Published 2011 Blackwell Publishing Ltd.

Sensory nerve conduction

Nerve and site	Peak latency	Amplitude	Segment	Latency difference	Distance	Conduction velocity
Sural.L						
Point B	NR ms	μV	Lateral malleolus-Point B	ms	mm	m/s
Sural.R						
Point B	NR ms	μV	Lateral malleolus-Point B	ms	mm	m/s
Median.L						
Digit II	3.8 ms	9 μV	Wrist-Digit II	3.8 ms	130 mm	49 m/s
Ulnar.L						
V Digit	3.5 ms	4 μV	Wrist-V Digit	2.5 ms	120 mm	40 m/s
Radial.L						
Forearm	2.8 ms	18 μV	Dorsum of hand-Forearm	2.7 ms	150 mm	51 m/s

Needle EMG examination

Muscle	Insertional	+Wave	Fibs	Fasc	Activator	Rate	Duration	Amplitude	Config	Other
	Insertional	Spontaneous activity			Volitional MUAPs					
Tibialis anterior.L	Normal	None	None	None	None	Normal	Normal	Normal	Normal	Normal
Gastrocnemius (Medial head.L)	Normal	None	None	None	None	Normal	Normal	Normal	Normal	Normal

Motor nerve conduction

Nerve and site	Latency	Amplitude	Distance	Conduction velocity
Peroneal.L				
Ankle	3.6 ms	1.4 mV	mm	m/s
Fibula (head)	14.2 ms	0.5 mV	280 mm	26 m/s
Popliteal fossa	16.5 ms	0.4 mV	100 mm	43 m/s
Tibial.L				
Ankle	4.7 ms	1.4 mV	mm	m/s
Tibial.R				
Ankle	4.4 ms	1.3 mV	mm	m/s
Peroneal.R				
Ankle	4.3 ms	1.8 mV	mm	m/s
Fibula (head)	13.2 ms	1.4 mV	290 mm	33 m/s
Popliteal fossa	15.2 ms	1.3 mV	80 mm	40 m/s
Median.L				
Wrist	3.2 ms	6.8 mV	mm	m/s
Antecubital	8.4 ms	4.9 mV	230 mm	48 m/s
Ulnar.L				
Wrist	3.2 ms	1.8 mV	mm	43 m/s

capsaicin and anti-inflammatory therapies, tramadol, and opioid therapy may be considered. The effect of HAART remains unclear.

NCVs: Bilateral sural sensory responses are absent and the left ulnar sensory nerve action potential amplitude is reduced. Left median and radial sensory responses are normal, but both peroneal and tibial compound motor action potential amplitudes are reduced. Left ulnar and median motor studies are normal. Thus, electrodiagnostic stud-

ies show a length-dependent, symmetric, sensorimotor polyneuropathy with predominantly axonal features.

REFERENCES:

1. Martin C, Solders G, Sonnerborg A, Hansson P. Antiretroviral therapy may improve sensory function in HIV-infected patients: A pilot study. *Neurology* 2000;54:2120.
2. Pomerantz R. Residual HIV-1 disease in the era of highly active antiretroviral therapy. *N Engl J Med* 1999;340:1672.

66. Slowly progressive leg and arm weakness— radiculopathy, plexopathy, ALS, or CIDP/AMN?

CLINICAL CASE: A 45-year-old man had 2 years of progressive right leg weakness. Over the past year he has begun to trip. Months ago, his right arm began to weaken without pain or sensory loss. Examination showed mild weakness (4+/5 MRC) of the right foot eversion and dorsiflexion; mild weakness (5−/5) of the right thenar muscles; fasciculations in the right quadriceps, and no right brachioradialis, biceps and ankle reflexes. All other reflexes, sensory testing, creatine kinase, complete blood count and metabolic panel, brain and cervical/lumbar spine MRI were normal. Anti-GM1 antibody titers were high.

DIFFERENTIAL DIAGNOSIS: The clinical diagnosis might include amyotrophic lateral sclerosis (ALS), radiculopathy, plexopathy, multifocal motor neuropathy (MMN), a chronic inflammatory demyelinating polyradiculoneuropathy (CIDP), Lewis-Sumner syndrome (MADSAM), mononeuritis multiplex hereditary motor sensory neuropathy type 2, a hereditary neuropathy with liability to pressure palsies, or a toxic neuropathy. The electromyography (EMG) findings, asymmetrical weakness, and reduced reflexes in the affected nerves exclude a myopathy. The lack of sensory deficit suggests ALS or MMN. Multifocal motor neuropathy—MMN (or multifocal motor neuropathy with conduction block)—is characterized by lower motor neuron signs. The absence of upper motor neuron sign, acute denervations in only affected myotomes, and the presence of conduction block argue against ALS.

DIAGNOSIS AND COMMENTS: Multifocal motor neuropathy. Motor nerve conduction studies in MMN often show evidence of conduction block, representing focal demyelination. Sensory conduction through the same segment of nerve is normal. Elevated titers of anti-GM1 antibodies are evident in 70–80% of patients with MNN. While conduction blocks may be seen in demyelinating neuropathies such as CIDP, the normal sensory responses point toward a diagnosis of MMN [1]. MMN with conduction block is an acquired immune-mediated demyelinating neuropathy with slowly progressive weakness, wrist drop, grip weakness, impaired dexterity, foot drop, fasciculations, and cramping, without significant sensory involvement. Weakness is a result of nerve conduction block, usually the radial, common peroneal, median, or ulnar nerves. MMN may resemble ALS, but muscle atrophy, bulbar symptoms, and more rapid progression are often not seen in MMN. Elevated anti-GM1 antibody titers occur in 50% of patients with MMN. Unlike ALS, MMN usually responds to intravenous immunoglobulin (IVIg) or cyclophosphamide, even after onset of symptoms [2, 3]. Anecdotal reports suggest that rituximab, interferon-β, azathioprine, and cyclosporine may be efficacious.

PROGNOSIS: Usually good with 70–80% of patients responding to treatment with intravenous immunoglobulin or cyclophosphamide, even after many years [4]. Unresponding patients may experience only slowly progressive weakness, with more than 90% of patients remaining employed.

Clinical Electrophysiology. By © Peter W. Kaplan and Thien Nguyen.
Published 2011 Blackwell Publishing Ltd.

Sensory nerve conduction

Nerve and site	Peak latency	Amplitude	Segment	Latency difference	Distance	Conduction velocity
Sural.R						
Point B	3.2 ms	10 µV	Lateral malleolus-Point B	2.2 ms	105 mm	48 m/s
Sural.R						
Point B	3.1 ms	9 µV	Lateral malleolus-Point B	2.1 ms	105 mm	48 m/s
Median.R						
Wrist	4.1 ms	17 µV	Digit II (index finger)-Wrist	2.5 ms	130 mm	52 m/s
Ulnar.R						
Wrist	3.1 ms	11 µV	Digit V (little finger)-Wrist	2.1 ms	110 mm	50 m/s
Radial.R						
Forearm	1.7 ms	26 µV	Dorsum of hand-Forearm	1.7 ms	100 mm	59 m/s

Motor nerve conduction

Nerve and site	Latency	Amplitude	Segment	Latency difference	Distance	Conduction velocity
Peroneal.R						
Ankle	5.4 ms	2.1 mV	EDP-Ankle	5.4 ms	mm	m/s
Fibular Head	13.2 ms	2.0 mV	Ankle-Fibular Head	7.8 ms	310 mm	40 m/s
Pop Fossa	15.2 ms	1.1 mV	Fibular Head-Pop Fossa	2.0 ms	90 mm	45 m/s
Tibial.R						
ankle	4.7 ms	14.5 mV	AH-ankle	4.7 ms	mm	m/s
Tibial.L						
ankle	4.6 ms	16.9 mV	AH-ankle	4.6 ms	mm	m/s
Peroneal.L						
Ankle	5.3 ms	4.3 mV	EDB-Ankle	5.3 ms	mm	m/s
Fibular Head	12.8 ms	4.3 mV	Ankle-Fibular Head	7.5 ms	310 mm	41 m/s
Pop Fossa	14.2 ms	3.8 mV	Fibular Head-Pop Fossa	1.4 ms	100 mm	71 m/s
Median.L						
wrist	3.0 ms	4.4 mV	APB-wrist	3.0 ms	mm	m/s
antecubital	7.6 ms	1.4 mV	wrist-antecubital	4.6 ms	250 mm	54 m/s
Ulnar.L						
wrist	3.0 ms	3.8 mV	wrist	3.0 ms	mm	m/s

Needle EMG examination

Motor NCS Median-APS

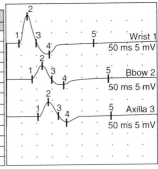

Muscle	Insertional	+ Wave	Fibs	Fasc	Activation	Rate	Duration	Amplitude	Config	Other
	Insertional	**Spontaneous activity**					**Volitional MUAPs**			
Peroneus longus.R	Normal	+2	+2	None	MD	Rapid	SI	SI	Normal	
Tibialis anterior.R	Normal	+3	+3	None	GD	Rapid	SI	SI		
Gastrocnemius.R	Normal	None	None	None						
Rectus femoris.R	Normal	None	None	None			Normal	Normal	Normal	Normal
Iliopsoas.R	Normal	None	None	None						
L5-paraspinous.R	Normal	None	None	None			Normal	Normal	Normal	Normal
Gastrocnemius.L	Normal	None	None	None						
Abductor pollicis br. R	Normal	+3	+3	None	GD	Rapid	SI	SI		
Pronator teres.R	Normal	+3	+3	None	GD	Rapid	SI	SI		
First dorsal intero.R	Normal	None	None	None			Normal	Normal	Normal	Normal
Biceps.R	Normal	None	None	None						
Deltoid.R	Normal	None	None	None			Normal	Normal	Normal	Normal
Abductor pollicis br.L	Normal	None	None	None						

NCVs: Sensory nerve action potentials are normal. There are multiple conduction blocks in the right median nerve in the forearm and right peroneal nerve above the knee. Concentric needle EMG examination shows acute denervation (i.e., fibrillations and positive sharp waves) in the right upper and lower limbs. There are also reduced (neurogenic) recruitment and voluntary motor units with long duration and large amplitude; many are polyphasic. In summary, there are multifocal motor neuropathies with conduction blocks.

REFERENCES:

1. Chaudhry V, Corse AM, Cornblath DR, Kuncl RW, Freimer ML, Griffin JW. Multifocal motor neuropathy: Electrodiagnostic features. *Muscle Nerve* Feb 1994;17(2):198–205.

2. Nobile-Orazio E, Cappellari A, Priori A. Multifocal motor neuropathy: Current concepts and controversies. *Muscle Nerve* 2005;31(6):663–680.

3. Hughes RA. European federation of neurological societies/peripheral nerve society guideline on management of multifocal motor neuropathy. Report of a joint task force of the European federation of neurological societies and the peripheral nerve society. *J Peripher Nerv Syst* 2006;11(1):1–8.

4. Felice KJ, Goldstein JM. Monofocal motor neuropathy: Improvement with intravenous immunoglobulin. *Muscle Nerve* 2002;25(5):674–678.

67. Progressive thigh pain and leg weakness—radiculopathy, vasculitis, neuropathy, or amyotrophy?

CLINICALCASE: An 82-year-old woman had worsening right thigh pain over 2 weeks, followed by right leg weakness and difficulty walking. She had diabetes mellitus. Examination showed weakness in the right quadriceps (4+/5 MRC), of right thigh adduction (4/5), and hip flexion (4+/5) only. Reflexes were 1/4 in the right knee only. There was normal body and limb sensation; normal creatine kinase, complete blood count, and metabolic panel; normal brain and lumbar spine MRI, and no fever.

DIFFERENTIAL DIAGNOSIS: The differential diagnosis includes compressive radiculopathy, ischemic lumbar plexopathy, vasculitis, lumbar spondylolysis and spondylolisthesis, or less commonly cauda equina syndrome, mononeuritis multiplex, or neoplastic lumbosacral plexopathy. Some of these findings occur with postpolio syndrome, radiation-induced lumbosacral plexopathy, and obstetric–gynecologic complications or complications following any pelvic surgery. Sensory loss and diminished reflexes suggest a peripheral nervous system process. Quadriceps muscle, thigh adduction, and hip flexion weaknesses exclude a femoral neuropathy, but point to-

ward either a radiculopathy or plexopathy. The absent knee reflexes correspond to an L4 nerve roots and/or plexus lesion. Electromyography (EMG) showing acute denervation in L2–L4 paraspinous muscles and other L2–L4 innervated myotomes suggests a plexoradiculopathy. The most common type of diabetic polyradiculopathy involving high lumbar radiculopathy involving the L2, L3, and L4 roots is a syndrome called diabetic amyotrophy.

DIAGNOSIS AND COMMENT: The patient has diabetic amyotrophy [1]. Diabetic amyotrophy carries a good prognosis with functional recovery in 12–24 months in 60% of patients [2, 3]. Mild weakness, discomfort, and stiffness often persist for years. Occasional relapses occur. Management is directed at good glycemic control. Intravenous human immunoglobulin (IVIg) [4], cyclophosphamide, and methylprednisolone may improve some patients, but are controversial [4]. Neurologic recovery may be slow, and physical therapy can improve functional mobility (e.g., transfers and ambulation), the use of assistive devices, and to avoid contractures.

Clinical Electrophysiology. By © Peter W. Kaplan and Thien Nguyen. Published 2011 Blackwell Publishing Ltd.

Sensory nerve conduction

Nerve and site	Peak latency	Amplitude	Segment	Latency difference	Distance	Conduction velocity
Sural.L						
Point B	NR ms	µV	Lateral malleolus-Point B	ms	mm	m/s
Sural.R						
Point B	NR ms	µV	Lateral malleolus-Point B	ms	mm	m/s
Median.L						
Digit II	3.8 ms	8 µV	Wrist-Digit II	3.8 ms	130 mm	49 m/s
Ulnar.L						
V. Digit	3.5 ms	3 µV	Wrist-V Digit	2.5 ms	120 mm	40 m/s
Radial.L						
Forearm	2.8 ms	15 µV	Dorsum of hand-Forearm	2.7 ms	150 mm	51 m/s
Saphenous.R						
Media Tibia	NR ms	µV	Medial Malleolus-Medial Tibia	ms	mm	0 m/s
Saphenous.L						
Media Tibia	2.8 ms	4 µV	Medial Malleolus-Medial Tibia	2.8 ms	110 mm	m/s

Motor nerve conduction

Nerve and site	Latency	Amplitude	Distance	Conduction velocity
Peroneal.L				
Ankle	3.6 ms	1.4 mV	mm	m/s
Fibula (head)	14.2 ms	0.5 mV	280 mm	26 m/s
Popliteal fossa	16.5 ms	0.4 mV	100 mm	43 m/s
Tibial.L				
Ankle	4.7 ms	1.4 mV	mm	m/s
Tibial.R				
Ankle	4.4 ms	1.3 mV	mm	m/s
Peroneal.R				
Ankle	4.3 ms	1.8 mV	mm	m/s
Fibula (head)	13.2 ms	1.4 mV	290 mm	33 m/s
Popliteal fossa	15.2 ms	1.3 mV	80 mm	40 m/s
Median.L				
Wrist	3.2 ms	6.8 mV	mm	m/s
Antecubital	8.4 ms	4.9 mV	230 mm	48 m/s
Ulnar.L				
Wrist	3.2 ms	1.8 mV	mm	43 m/s

Needle EMG examination

Muscle	Insertional	Spontaneous activity			Volitional MUAPs					Other
	Insertional	+Wave	Fibs	Fasc	Activation	Rate	Duration	Amplitude	Config	
Vastus lateralis.R	Increased	+3	+3	None	GD	Rapid	Normal	Normal	Normal	
Rectus femoris.R	Increased	+2	+2	None	GD	Rapid	Normal	Normal	Normal	
Iliopsoas.R	Increased	+2	+2	None	MD	Normal	SI	SI	Polyphasic	
Thigh adductor.R	Increased	+2	+2	None	MD	Normal	SI	SI	Polyphasic	
Med gastrocnemius.R	Normal	None	None	None	Normal	Normal	Normal	Normal	Normal	
Gluteus medium.R	Increased	+2	+2	None	MD	Normal	SI	SI	Polyphasic	
L3-paraspinous.R	Increased	+2	+2	None	MD	Normal	SI	SI	Polyphasic	
Vastus lateralis.L	Normal	None	None	None	Normal	Normal	Normal	Normal	Normal	

NCVs: The sensory and motor distal latencies, conduction velocities, and F-wave latencies in the upper and lower extremities are slow. Right femoral compound motor action potential amplitude is reduced, and both saphenous sensory responses are absent. Concentric needle EMG examination showed acute denervation (i.e., fibrillations and positive sharp waves) in the right quadriceps, thigh adductors, iliopsoas, and L2–L4 paraspinous muscles. There are reduced (neurogenic) recruitment and long duration, large-amplitude polyphasic motor units.

REFERENCES:

1. Garland H. Diabetic amyotrophy. *Br Med J* 1955;2(4951): 1287–1290.
2. Asbury AK. Proximal diabetic neuropathy. *Ann Neurol* 1977;2(3):179–180.
3. Dyck PJ, Windebank AJ. Diabetic and nondiabetic lumbosacral radiculoplexus neuropathies: New insights into pathophysiology and treatment. *Muscle Nerve* 2002;25(4):477–491.
4. Kawagashira Y, Watanabe H, Oki Y, Iijima M, Koike H, Hattori H, Katsuno M, Tanaka F, Sobue G. Intravenous immunoglobulin therapy markedly ameliorates muscle weakness and severe pain in proximal diabetic neuropathy. *J Neurol Neurosurg Psychiatry* 2007;78(8):899–901.

Index

Acute intermittent porphyria (AIP), diagnosis and treatment of
  case study on, 162
  diagnosis, 162, 164
  EMG/nerve conduction studies, 163, 165
  treatment, 164
Acute polyneuropathies, 162
Akinetic mutism, 77
Alcohol abuse. *See* Low-voltage fast beta pattern
Alpha coma
  ancillary testing, 20
  clinical correlation, 20
  clinical evaluation, 20
  differential diagnosis, 20
  EEG recording, 21
  etiology, 20
  prognosis, 20
  treatment, 20
Alpha frequency patterns (AFPs), 20–21
ALS. *See* Amyotrophic lateral sclerosis (ALS)
Altered mental status, definition of, 1
Amyotrophic lateral sclerosis (ALS), 122, 174
  ancillary testing, 122
  clinical correlates, 122
  clinical evaluation, 122
  differential diagnosis, 122
  nerve conduction studies, 123
  prognosis, 122
  treatment, 122–3
Anesthetic agent, in SE, 61–2, 64, 66
Anoxic coma, prognostic value of SSEP in
  ancillary testing, 92
  clinical correlates, 92
  clinical evaluation, 92
  differential diagnosis, 92
  etiology, 92
  prognosis, 92–3
Antiepileptic drugs, 14
Anti-epileptic drugs (AEDs), 30, 40
  BIPLEDs and, 44
  and frontal lobe seizures, 52
  and occipital lobe seizures, 58
  parietal lobe partial seizures and, 56

  in PLEDs, 40
  in simple partial status epilepticus, 66, 68
  temporal lobe seizures and, 54

Babinski reflexes, in hypoglycemia, 32
Baclofen, 28
Baclofen toxicity
  ancillary testing, 28
  clinical correlation, 28
  clinical evaluation, 28
  differential diagnosis, 28
  EEG pattern, 29
  etiology, 28
  prognosis, 28
  treatment, 28
Benzodiazepine, 4, 28, 40, 44, 61–2, 66, 68, 82, 155
Beta, diffuse and frontal fast activity
  ancillary testing, 4
  clinical correlates, 4
  clinical evaluation, 4
  differential diagnosis, 4
  EEG pattern, 5
  etiology, 4
  medication effect and, 5
  prognosis, 4
Beta frequency bands, 5
Bicuculline-insensitive GABA-B receptors, 28
Bilateral independent PLEDs (BIPLEDs)
  ancillary testing, 44
  clinical correlates, 44
  definition, 44
  differential diagnosis, 44
  EEG recording, 45
  etiology, 44
  frequency of discharges, 44
  prognosis, 44
  treatment, 44
Botulism, diagnosis and treatment of
  case study on, 166–8
Brachial plexopathy
  ancillary testing, 128
  clinical correlates, 128

Brachial plexopathy (*cont.*)
  clinical evaluation, 128
  differential diagnosis, 128
  needle EMG examination, 129
  nerve conduction studies, 128
  prognosis, 128
  treatment, 128
Brainstem auditory evoked potentials (BAEPs), 94, 97
  in worsening hearing, 110–11
Burst/suppression
  ancillary testing, 26
  clinical correlate, 26
  clinical evaluation, 26
  differential diagnosis, 26
  EEG pattern, 27
  etiology, 26
  prognosis, 26
  treatment, 26

Catatonia, 73, 82, 84, 88, 91, 154
  ancillary testing, 90
  clinical correlates, 90
  clinical evaluation, 90
  differential diagnosis, 90
  EEG recording, 91
  etiology, 90
Closed head injury (CHI), 94
Coma, 76, 82, 84, 88, 90, 152, 154
  EEG of, 77–8
  Glasgow coma scale, 75
Comatose patients, 62, 64, 68, 70–71, 75, 97, 110
Complex partial status epilepticus (CPSE), 64
  of frontal region. *See* Complex partial status epilepticus, frontal
  of temporal region. *See* Complex partial status epilepticus, temporal
Complex partial status epilepticus, frontal
  ancillary testing, 62
  clinical correlates, 62
  clinical evaluation, 62
  differential diagnosis, 62
  EEG pattern, 63
  etiology, 62
  prognosis, 62
  treatment, 62
Complex partial status epilepticus, temporal
  ancillary testing, 64
  clinical correlates, 64
  clinical evaluation, 64
  differential diagnosis, 64
  EEG pattern, 65
  etiology, 64
  prognosis, 64
  treatment, 64
Compound muscle action potential (CMAP), 166
Confusion, definition of, 1

Consciousness
  arousal, 76
  awareness, 76
  definition of, 76
Convulsive status epilepticus (CSE), 61
Critical illness neuromyopathy
  ancillary testing, 124
  clinical correlates, 124
  clinical evaluation, 124
  differential diagnosis, 124
  needle EMG, 125
  nerve conduction studies, 126
  prognosis, 124
  treatment, 124

Delirium, definition of, 1
Delta, diffuse and slow activity
  ancillary testing, 8
  clinical correlation, 8
  clinical evaluation, 8
  differential diagnosis, 8
  EEG pattern, 9–10
  etiology, 8
  prognosis, 8
Diabetic amyotrophy, diagnosis and treatment of
  case study on, 178–80
Distal symmetric peripheral neuropathy (DSPN). *See* HIV-related DSPN, diagnosis and treatment of

EEG, 2, 88, 90
  alpha coma, 21
  anoxic coma, 79
  baclofen toxicity, 29
  BIPLEDs, 44–5
  bursts of epileptiform activity with suppression periods, 27
  coma, 77–8
  diffuse alpha activity in comma, 21
  frontal intermittent delta activity, 13
  frontal lobe seizures, 52–3
  generalized suppression with no cortical activity, 25
  hypoglycemia, 33
  in LIS, 78, 83
  lithium toxicity, 31
  low-voltage fast beta pattern, 19
  medium- to high-voltage diffuse fast beta pattern, 5
  occipital blindness and seizures, 150
  occipital intermittent rhythmic delta activity, 15
  occipital lobe seizures, 59
  parietal lobe seizures, 57
  PLEDs, 40–41
  slow delta activity, 10
  spindle coma, 23
  temporal lobe seizures, 55
  theta activity, 5
  triphasic waves, 17
  for VS, 78, 84–5
  widespread arrhythmic delta pattern, 9

Electrocerebral inactivity, 25
Electromyography (EMG), 114, 124, 130
EMG. *See* Electromyography (EMG)
Encephalopathy, definition of, 1
Epilepsia partialis continua, 52, 62
Epilepsy monitoring, 49
EPs. *See* Evoked potentials (EPs)
Evoked potentials (EPs), 97
    brainstem auditory evoked potentials, 97
    role in coma prognosis, 78
    somatosensory evoked potentials, 97
    visual evoked potentials, 97
    in VS patients, 78, 84
Eye blink artifact, 7
Eye deviation, 68–9
Eye leads, 12–13
Eye movement artifact, and FIRDA, 12–13

Femoral neuropathy
    ancillary testing, 130
    clinical correlates, 130
    clinical evaluation, 130
    differential diagnosis, 130
    etiology, 130
    needle EMG examination, 131
    nerve conduction studies, 130–31
    treatment, 130
Focal arrhythmic (polymorphic) delta activity
    ancillary testing, 36
    clinical correlates, 36
    clinical evaluation, 36
    definition, 36
    differential diagnosis, 36
    EEG pattern, 37
    etiology, 36
Frontal glioma with complex partial seizures, case study on,
        156–7
Frontal intermittent rhythmic delta activity
        (FIRDA)
    ancillary testing, 12
    clinical correlates of, 12
    clinical evaluation, 12
    differential diagnosis, 12
    EEG pattern, 13
    in elderly patients, 12
    etiology, 12
    and eye movement artifact, 12–13
    prognosis, 12
Frontal lobe partial seizures
    ancillary testing, 52
    clinical correlates, 52
    clinical evaluation, 52
    differential diagnosis, 52
    EEG recording, 53
    etiology, 52
    prognosis, 52
    treatment, 52

Functional magnetic resonance imaging (fMRI), 76–7,
        82
    comma, 78
    MCS, 77
    responses to language stimuli, study of, 79

Gait and posture testing, 114
Generalized nonconvulsive status epilepticus (GNSE), 64, 70,
        158
    clinical correlates, 70
    clinical evaluation, 70
    differential diagnosis, 70
    EEG recording, 71–2
    etiology, 70
    prognosis, 70
    treatment, 70
Generalized periodic epileptiform discharges (GPEDs), 46–7
    ancillary testing, 46
    clinical correlates, 46
    clinical evaluation, 46
    differential diagnosis, 46
    EEG recording, 47
    etiology, 46
    prognosis, 46
    treatment, 46
Glasgow coma scale, 20, 22, 26, 70, 75, 82, 84, 92, 94, 152
GNSE. *See* Generalized nonconvulsive status epilepticus (GNSE)
Guillain-Barré syndrome (GBS)
    ancillary testing, 136
    clinical correlates, 136
    clinical evaluation, 136
    differential diagnosis, 136
    EMG/nerve conduction study, 137–8
    prognosis, 136
    treatment, 136

Head trauma, prognostic value of SSEP in
    ancillary testing, 94
    clinical considerations, 94
    clinical correlates, 94
    clinical evaluation, 94
    differential diagnosis, 94
    prognosis, 94–5
HIV-related DSPN, diagnosis and treatment of
    case study on, 170
Hollow skull phenomenon, 78
Hypoglycemia
    ancillary testing, 32
    clinical correlates, 32
    clinical evaluation, 32
    differential diagnosis, 32
    EEG pattern, 33
    etiology, 32
    prognosis, 32
    treatment, 32

Index of global cortical function, determination of, 79

Limbic encephalopathy
    ancillary testing, 34
    clinical correlates, 34
    clinical evaluation, 34
    differential diagnosis, 34
    EEG pattern, 35
    etiology, 34
Limbic status epilepticus from mycoplasma pneumonia, case
        study on, 154–5
LIS. See Locked-in syndrome (LIS)
Lithium toxicity
    ancillary testing, 30
    clinical correlates, 30
    clinical evaluation, 30
    differential diagnosis, 30
    EEG pattern in, 31
    etiology, 30
    prognosis, 30
    treatment, 30
Locked-in syndrome (LIS), 73, 75, 84, 88, 90, 152,
        154
    ancillary testing, 82
    clinical correlates, 82
    clinical evaluation, 82
    definition of, 77
    differential diagnosis, 82
    EEG of, 78
    EEG recording, 83
    PET findings in, 78
    prognosis, 83
    treatment, 83
Long-latency auditory responses (N70), 78
Lorazepam, 16, 28, 30, 46, 61, 64, 68, 70
Low-voltage fast beta pattern
    ancillary testing, 18
    clinical correlates, 18
    clinical evaluation, 18
    differential diagnosis, 18
    EEG recording, 19
    etiology, 18
    prognosis, 18
Low-voltage suppressed pattern
    ancillary testing, 24
    clinical correlation, 24
    clinical evaluation, 24
    differential diagnosis, 24
    EEG report with no cortical activity, 25
    etiology, 24
    prognosis, 24
Lumbar radiculopathy
    ancillary testing, 134
    clinical correlates, 134
    clinical evaluation, 134
    differential diagnosis, 134
    EMG/nerve conduction study, 134–5
    prognosis, 134
    treatment, 134

Minimally conscious state (MCS), 73, 75–7
    ancillary testing, 88
    clinical correlates, 88
    clinical evaluation, 88
    definition of, 76
    differential diagnosis, 88
    EEG recordings, 89
    etiology, 88
    and fMRI findings, 76–7
    prognosis, 88
    treatment, 88–9
Multifocal motor neuropathy (MMN), diagnosis and treatment
        of
    case study on, 174–6
Muscle artifact, 9, 57, 67
Muscle testing, 113
Myasthenia gravis (MG)
    ancillary testing, 140
    clinical correlates, 140
    clinical evaluation, 140
    differential diagnosis, 140
    EMG/nerve conduction study, 140–41, 143–4
    etiology, 140
    treatment, 140
Myositis
    ancillary testing, 142
    clinical correlates, 142
    clinical evaluation, 142
    differential diagnosis, 142
    prognosis, 142
    treatment, 143

NCSE. See Nonconvulsive status epilepticus (NCSE)
Neuromuscular disorders, 113
    clinical evaluation of, 116
    diagnosing of, 113–14
    in ICU patients, causes of, 115
    laboratory evaluation of, 117
    segmental weakness and sensory loss in, 119–20
    weakness in, 113
Neuromuscular junction dysfunction, 166. See also Botulism,
        diagnosis and treatment of
Neuropathic syndromes during HIV infection, 170
Nonconvulsive status epilepticus (NCSE), 1, 16, 28, 30, 61, 70,
        90, 158. See also Complex partial status epilepticus
        (CPSE)

Occipital blindness and seizures, case study on,
        150–51
Occipital epileptic activity, 68
Occipital intermittent rhythmic delta activity (OIRDA)
    ancillary testing, 14
    in children, 14
    clinical correlates, 14
    clinical evaluation, 14
    EEG pattern, 15
    etiology, 14

prognosis, 14
treatment, 14
Occipital lobe simple partial seizures
ancillary testing, 58
clinical correlates, 58
clinical evaluation, 58
differential diagnosis, 58
EEG recording in, 59
etiology, 58
prognosis, 58
treatment, 58
Organ dysfunction
and diffuse slow theta activity, 6–7

Paralysis and respiratory failure in the ICU, causes of, 115
Parietal lobe simple partial seizures
ancillary testing, 56
clinical correlates, 56
clinical evaluation, 56
differential diagnosis, 56
EEG pattern, 57
etiology, 56
prognosis, 56
treatment, 56
Periodic discharges (PDs), 39
Permanent VS, 77, 85
Persistent vegetative state (PVS), 26, 73, 77, 85, 97
Phenytoin, 61
PLEDs. See Pseudoperiodic lateralized epileptiform discharges
(PLEDs)
Positron emission tomography (PET), 34, 54, 56, 66, 83
LIS and, 78
Posterior reversible encephalopathy syndrome (PRES), 150
Potassium channel antibody-associated encephalopathy
(VGKC), case study on, 160–61
Prolonged unresponsiveness, states of, 73, 76–7
behavioral characteristics in, 77
electrophysiological findings, 77–8
functional imaging, role of, 78–9
prognosis using electrophysiology, 79
Pseudoperiodic lateralized epileptiform discharges (PLEDs)
ancillary testing, 40
clinical correlates, 40
clinical evaluation, 40
definition, 40
differential diagnosis, 40
EEG recording, 41
etiology, 40
frequency of discharges, 40
prognosis, 40
treatment, 40–41

Riluzole, 123

Secondary generalization, 68
Segmental peripheral neurological disorders, evaluation of,
120

Seizures, 49
complex partial, 52, 54, 56
and EEG, 49–50
frontal lobe seizures, 52–3
in occipital lobes, 58–9
parietal lobe seizures, 56–7
partial seizures, 49
and PLEDs, 39. See also Pseudoperiodic lateralized
epileptiform discharges (PLEDs)
simple partial seizure, 54, 56
temporal lobe seizures, 54–5
Sensory neuropathy/ganglionopathy
ancillary testing, 132
clinical correlates, 132
clinical evaluation, 132
differential diagnosis, 132
needle EMG examination, 133
nerve conduction studies, 132
prognosis, 132
Short-latency auditory evoked potentials, 77
Simple partial status epilepticus, occipital
ancillary testing, 68
clinical correlates, 68
clinical evaluation, 68
differential diagnosis, 68
EEG recording, 69
etiology, 68
prognosis, 68
treatment, 68
Simple partial status epilepticus, parietal
ancillary testing, 66
clinical correlates, 66
clinical evaluation, 66
differential diagnosis, 66
EEG recording, 67
etiology, 66
prognosis, 66
treatment, 66
Somatosensory evoked potentials (SSEPs), 2, 8, 20, 22, 26, 46,
78–9, 92, 97
after prolonged cardiac arrest
clinical case study, 104
responses above brachial plexus, absence of, 104–5
in asystolic cardiac arrest
clinical case study, 102
SSEP cortical responses, absence of, 102–3
in diffuse cortical anoxic injury
clinical case study, 100
cortical and subcortical responses, absence of, 100–101
median and tibial nerve SSEP, after traumatic spinal cord
injury, 106–7
in midbrain lesion
clinical case study, 98
cortical responses, absence of, 98–9
Spindle beta patterns, in children, 4
Spindle coma
ancillary testing, 22

Spindle coma (*cont.*)
   clinical correlation, 22
   clinical evaluation, 22
   differential diagnosis, 22
   EEG pattern, 23
   etiology, 22
   prognosis, 22
   treatment, 22
SSEPs. *See* Somatosensory evoked potentials (SSEPs)
Static encephalopathies
   and diffuse slow theta activity, 6–7
Statin-induced myopathy
   ancillary testing, 146
   clinical correlates, 146
   clinical evaluation, 146
   differential diagnosis, 146
   EMG/nerve conduction studies, 147–8
   prognosis, 146
   treatment, 146
Status epilepticus (SE), 49, 61. *See also* Nonconvulsive status
     epilepticus (NCSE)
   frontal lobe CPSE, 62–3
   generalized nonconvulsive status epilepticus, 70–72
   occipital lobe simple partial SE, 68–9
   parietal lobe simple partial SE, 66–7
   temporal lobe CPSE, 64–5

Temporal lobe partial seizures
   ancillary testing, 54
   clinical correlates, 54
   clinical evaluation, 54
   differential diagnosis, 54
   EEG pattern, 55
   etiology, 54
   prognosis, 54
   treatment, 54
Theta, diffuse slow activity
   ancillary testing, 6
   clinical correlates, 6

clinical evaluation, 6
differential diagnosis, 6
EEG pattern, 7
etiology, 6
prognosis, 6
Thigh pain and leg weakness. *See* Diabetic amyotrophy,
     diagnosis and treatment of
Tonic–clonic seizure, 14
Toxic encephalopathy. *See* Baclofen toxicity
Triphasic waves (TWs), 16, 28, 44, 64, 70, 158
   ancillary testing, 16
   baclofen overdose and, 28–9
   clinical correlates, 16
   clinical evaluation, 16
   differential diagnosis, 16
   EEG pattern, 17
   etiology, 16
   lithium toxicity and, 30–31
   prognosis, 16
   treatment, 16
TWs. *See* Triphasic waves (TWs)

Unresponsiveness, case study on states of, 152–3. *See also*
     Locked-in syndrome (LIS)

Valproate-induced hyperammonemia, case study on, 158–9
Vegetative state (VS), 73, 75, 77, 82, 90, 152, 154
   ancillary testing, 84
   clinical correlates, 84
   clinical evaluation, 84
   differential diagnosis, 84–5
   EEG of, 78
   EEG recording, 85
   etiology, 84
   prognosis, 85
   treatment, 85
Visual evoked potentials (VEPs), 97
   in worsening vision, 108–9
VS. *See* Vegetative state (VS)